Praise for *Spiritual Genomics*

Fred's boundless curiosity and impeccable research connect the dots between exploration and science, giving us paths to follow to stay healthy, happy and spiritually expanding. His book is a must-read for those who seek new perspectives from the ancients to modern possibilities for shifting ourselves and our DNA.

— Jonette Crowley, Spiritual "Indiana Jones,"
author of *The Eagle and the Condor* and *Soul Body Fusion*

Wow! What an incredible book. I agree with Dr Grover in that the drug of choice in our chaotic world today is "stress" and getting back to the simple acts of mindfulness, sacred plant medicine and sacred geometry is a must, or our world will suffer greatly. There is so much good in this book and coming from an MD makes it even better.

— Daniel Gutierrez, international best-selling
author of *Radical Mindfulness* | Speaker | Mindful
Leadership Expert | Master Life/Business Coach

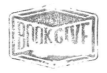

In this beautifully written book, Dr. Fred Grover shares discoveries from his lifelong, planetary odyssey to uncover the hidden connections between the material and energetic realms. The powerful techniques he suggests can change the expression of your genes to increase longevity and to stay healthier longer.

—Terry Grossman, MD, Grossman Wellness Center,
Denver / internationally recognized
Anti-Aging and Longevity Specialist

Fred Grover takes us on a journey through time and space to investigate different healing modalities in his search for discovering different ways to assist our health and happiness. A combination travel journal, scientific treatise, historical document and spiritual exploration, *Spiritual Genomics* is fascinating, covering topics as diverse as the healing abilities of sacred geometry, sound, water, dance, meditation, plant medicine and much more. This book is a cornucopia of knowledge, highlighting Dr. Grover's experiences as he learns and discovers various aspects of the healing process from many different traditions. Truly a good read.

— Jonathan Goldman, world famous musician,
author, and sound healer.

Dr. Grover has outdone himself in a heroic task of synthesizing an amazing work, revealing cutting edge research on perhaps the most interesting and important topics of our time—which our ancestors knew of and we are now collectively remembering at a whole new octave of understanding. He addresses the basis of frequency and vibration as the stratum underlying creation, which gives us many keys' to quantum evolutionary leaps—so essential for the times we live in.

—Kimba Arem, musician,
recording artist, author, sound healer.
www.gaearth.com / www.radiancehealth.com /
www.secretofwaterthemovie.com

Spiritual Genomics

Becky,

I hope you enjoy this exploration of science & spirituality!

Wishing you the best in health, wellness & spiritual growth.

Peace,

Fred

Spiritual Genomics

A physician's deep dive beyond modern medicine, discovering unique keys to optimizing DNA health, longevity, and happiness!

Fred Grover Jr., MD

Spiritual Genomics Press™
P.O. Box 202562
Denver 80220

Printed in the United States of America

For permission to reproduce parts of this book,
speaking engagement requests, or other questions,
please contact the author at fgroverjr@spiritualgenomics.com

Editor: Margaret A. Harrell, https://margaretharrell.com
Cover artwork: KA'ryna SH'ha, https://www.karynashha.com/her-story
Interior and cover design: Darlene Swanson, https://van-garde.com

Follow our Spiritual Genomics Facebook page!
Visit us at http://SpiritualGenomics.com

Publisher's Cataloging-In-Publication Data
(Prepared by The Donohue Group, Inc.)

Names: Grover, Fred, 1964- author.
Title: Spiritual genomics : a physician's deep dive beyond
modern medicine, discovering unique keys to optimizing
DNA health, longevity, and happiness! / Fred Grover Jr., M.D.

Description: Denver [Colorado] : Spiritual Genomics Press, [2019] |
Interest age level: 15 and up. | Includes bibliographical references.

Identifiers: ISBN 9781733772204 (pbk) | ISBN 9781733772211 (ebook)

Subjects: LCSH: Mental healing. | Alternative medicine. | Plants--Therapeutic use. |
Mind and body. | Health. | Grover, Fred, 1964---Philosophy.

Classification: LCC RZ400 .G76 2019 (print) |
LCC RZ400 (ebook) | DDC 615.8528--dc23

www.spiritualgenomics.com

Disclaimer

This book discusses a diverse number of therapies aimed at enhancing your health and genome beyond the typical topics in spirituality and medicine. That being said, there is a small section of this book (Chapter 8) which includes activities that should be discussed with your physician and overseen by a qualified medical practitioner in a safe and legal setting.

Furthermore, while this book does contain a discussion of psychoactive plants, including my own personal experimentation *in parts of the world where use of such plants is lawful,* most of the psychoactive plants discussed in this book remain unlawful under U.S. law. On no account should this book be read as a recommendation or advocacy to break U.S. law and certainly it should not be viewed as an endorsement for members of the medical community to counsel or recommend to their patients to use and experiment with psychoactive plants. Instead, the discussion is informational only, designed to promote further scientific research and advance the conversation around legalization of psychoactive plants for medical and therapeutic use. I am hopeful that all allopathic physicians, especially psychiatrists and primary care providers, will begin to appreciate the potential benefits of ancient healing modalities and the rapid growth of the public's interest in utilizing integrative, functional, and even shamanic medicine. I believe it's nonsensical that doctors are licensed to prescribe a host of highly addictive opioids produced for profit by the pharmaceutical industry, but are barred by law from working with naturally occurring psychoactive plants that have been used therapeutically by cultures indigenous to the Americas and elsewhere for millennia. We can only hope that physicians will start preventative treatment by incorporating remedies such as acupuncture, physical therapy, pulsed magnetic field therapy, light therapy, massage, etc., while more often recommending natural anti-inflammatories such as cucuminoids and CBD to help prevent the frequently unnecessary prescribing of an opioid, leading to further growth in the deadly epidemic.

Further, this book should not be read as an invitation to re-create or experiment with psychoactive materials—especially on your own. While I personally believe psychoactive plants hold medical and therapeutic promise, they should be used, if at all, only in lawful circumstances, preferably with qualified medical and therapeutic supervision and guidance, in the proper set and setting. While there is no tangible evidence that use of psychoactive plants has, in and of itself, killed anyone, there is always the risk of having a bad experience or unpleasant trip—an experience that can possibly have lasting psychological consequences, especially without proper integration.

Contents

Preface

The purpose of this book is to present unique opportunities to shift your DNA (genome) to a healthier state, thus benefiting your quality of life, happiness, and enhanced longevity potential. This is a book of light and love, and there is no darkness. I am not promoting or discouraging any religion; rather, I'm simply giving you creative tools to find your inner spiritual self as a means to improve your life. Whether your spirituality leads you to a god, a guru, an archangel, a pyramid, a tree, or a faraway galaxy, that's up to you.

I've written this from my heart over the last several years, with my own funding, on late nights and weekends while maintaining a busy private practice. Personal experiences of world travel, mindfulness-based processes, as well as knowledge obtained as a physician and clinician, are woven into this book. My hope is that it will inspire readers to personal growth, helping themselves and the planet.

What motivated me to put this out? Having been on this earth for over fifty years, I've observed our world trending toward an accelerated state of chaos and uncertainty, resulting in high degrees of individual stress, including a rising disconnect from one another and nature, as we've become overdependent on technology. Many other life forms are feeling a more dramatic effect, through extinction.

The greatest ancient civilizations reached climax states when they achieved high levels of fair civil governing, spirituality, art mastery, and architectural achievements, embracing a compassionate, understanding approach towards their neighbors. Those who learned to nurture the environment around them sustained themselves for longer periods of time, even during extended droughts.

As a physician focused on finding the root cause of illness, I'd like to hypothesize that the root cause of our current situation is greed, egocentrism, materialism, and a failure to draw on our deep spiritual self. This creates a blindness to the sacredness of those around us regardless of their race, country of origin, or social status. We must start with ourselves before we can heal the world, and we need to hurry up before it is too late. Politicians and religious leaders especially need to set selfish agendas behind and begin the pursuit towards oneness.

My introduction to the greeting "Namaste" was not at a trendy Denver yoga studio or seeing it as a bumper sticker on a Prius, but while being greeted by villagers in Nepal.

During my first volunteer medical trip to Nepal, in 1996, I asked the local organizer of the trip, Sajani, my friend and translator, "Why does every villager greet me with hands posed together, a smile, eye contact, and the word Namaste?" She replied, "Fred, they are saying they appreciate the god within you." I contemplated this for a moment after seeing several patients.

It was in this deep human connection that they accepted me, an outsider who could not speak their language. But they felt me through their hearts as I looked back in their eyes and said the ancient Sanskrit greeting, Namaste ("the divine in me bows to the divine in you"), with my hands together. My experience in the Himalayas shifted me in a way medical school and residency fell short. This book is my best effort to help you find or maintain your Namaste and to spread it to others with love!

To my critics who are not inspired by this book, please give it to someone who might be, recycle it, or burn it to warm your home.

To physicians looking for a large-scale evidence-based approach to mindfulness and spirituality, I point out that the National Institute of Health funding for mindfulness is minimal; the pharmaceutical industry will continue to dominate research, your lunches, your journals, and your meetings. Nevertheless, I found many significant studies free of pharmaceutical influence, supporting the benefits of mindfulness. Research citations are included to support the fact that we can change our DNA and brain structure with mindfulness and shifts towards a healthier, more balanced lifestyle.

I encourage readers to explore the possibilities of improving your health and longevity through these chapters, which range from simple mindfulness, sacred geometry, and sound healing to plant medicine in the jungles of Peru. I am grateful to the many experts in related fields for sharing their wisdom in interviews.

Wishing my readers a more meaningful, deep, passionate, loving, healthy, spiritual journey on Planet Earth.

FG

Chapter 1

The Asclepieion: Returning to the Wisdom of Ancient Healing

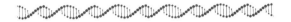

In the summer of 1996 my wife and I found ourselves at the sacred site of the asclepieion on the Greek island of Kos, the birthplace of Hippocrates, the "Father of Medicine" (c. 460–375 BC). He emerged amongst intellectual giants such as Sophocles, Socrates, and Democritus. But his medical teachings and therapies were often at odds with a belief in anthropomorphic deities—gods and goddesses, such as Apollo, Athena, and Zeus, who many Greeks believed could bring fearful pestilence and war, on the one hand, or peace and abundance, on the other. Oracles at Delphi and elsewhere were regularly consulted and seers for reading omens, such as in the flight of birds.[1]

Asclepius, "the Divine Physician," was the ancient god of medicine and healing to whom the Greeks (and Rome) set up sanctuaries. In mythology he was the son of Apollo but also of a mortal from Trikala, Thessaly. He first appeared in Homer's epic *The Iliad*, where he was not a god but a distinguished physician, a prince, whose two sons served as physician warriors in the battle of Troy. Asclepius learned medicine from the centaur Chiron. Somewhere down the line of centuries he acquired Apollo for a father. In Plato's *Phaedo*, Socrates's final words were in line with this tradition, "Crito, we ought to offer a cock to Asclepius. See to it, and don't forget."

The Sanctuary of Epidaurus, Greece, according to the UNESCO World Heritage website, is the first "organized sanatorium." It traces its healing practices to very ancient times:

> Initially, in the 2nd millennium BCE it was a site of ceremonial healing practices with curative associations that were later enriched through the cults of Apollo Maleatas in the 8th century BCE and then by Asklepios in the 6th century BCE. The Sanctuary of the two gods was developed into the single most important therapeutic center of the ancient world. These practices were subsequently spread to the rest of the Greco-Roman world and the Sanctuary thus became the cradle of medicine.

To a large extent the center diagnosed and healed through dream incubation—as was typical in the Asclepius cult.[2] Around 420 BC a similar sanctuary was set up in Athens. The temple to Asclepius in Rome was dedicated in 289 BC. Legend has it that because of a plague in Rome in 293 BC, a delegation went to Epidaurus to bring back a statue.

> The legend also relates that during the propitiatory rites a large serpent (one of the god's attributes) slithered from the sanctuary and hid in the Roman ship.

2

Certain that this was a sign of the god's favor, the Roman delegation quickly returned home, where the plague was still raging. As they were on the river Tiber and about to reach Rome, the snake crawled out of the ship and disappeared from sight on the island, marking the site where the temple was to be built. Work on the temple began immediately and it was dedicated in 289 BC—soon afterwards, the plague ended.[3]

Typically, healing in these clinic temples was overseen by priests (but primarily, the god himself in dreams).

When Hippocrates was born, there were already in or near Kos island two leading medical schools (or communities) supposedly descended from Podalirius—the son of Asclepius who survived the Trojan War. The reigning Cnidian branch believed disease should be treated according to the part of the body that was ill. Hippocrates, on the other hand, disagreed, "countering that the human body functioned as one unified organism, or *physis,* and must be treated, in health and disease, as one coherent, integrated whole."[4]

On his mother's side he was, by repute, descended from Heracles.[5] To us this sounds entirely like make-believe. But it's mixed with actual history, not to mention that in these long-ago centuries the world was not as rational as today.

As classical scholar Emma J. Edelstein and Johns Hopkins professor Ludwig Edelstein state in *Asclepius: Interpretation of the Testimonies*, his influence was so great that "in the final stages of paganism, of all genuinely Greek gods, [he] was judged the foremost antagonist of Christ."[6]

Not being able to teach at the multi-terraced Kos asclepieion (with its pools and fountains) I saw in ruins, as it was not yet built—although there is always the chance that excavations will turn up evidence that places it earlier—Hippocrates must have worked in a medical center located in the Old Town, Astypalaea, at the port where Club Med is today. The current town of Kos, built in 366/365 BC, is to the east. During his lifetime, presumably, construction on the Kos asclepieion complex I saw began, first as a simple altar; it took centuries to compete. How much of it he ever viewed is unknown, as at an indeterminate date, his children then grown, he spread his wings and relocated in the Thessaly region of Greece—leaving medical instruction at Kos in the charge of his protégé son in-law.[7]

But the doctors still there taught and healed after Hippocrates' methods.[8]

According to Jacques Jouanna in *Hippocrates*, the reputation of the Kos medical center "eclipsed" that of Cnidus.[9] Why did they pick this small island out in the Mediterranean to be one of their top "Mayo clinics"? I wondered, but it now seems fairly clear. Older and more celebrated, the Epidaurus asclepieion was supernaturally focused, delegating healing often to the gods.[10] But Kos had something else. It had the radical clinical approach of Hippocrates.

Are there energetic alignments here, or perhaps a history of being a healing center that preceded the Greeks by thousands of years?

Put another way, was the Kos asclepieion built on a site sacred earlier? Yes. It was built around a preexistent altar to Asclepius nearby to a temple to Apollo Cyparissus in a sacred cypress grove. By

4

myth Apollo loved a boy, Cyparissus, who accidentally killed his favorite stag and in grief found himself turned into a cypress tree. But recent excavations hint its sacred use goes back even further.[11]

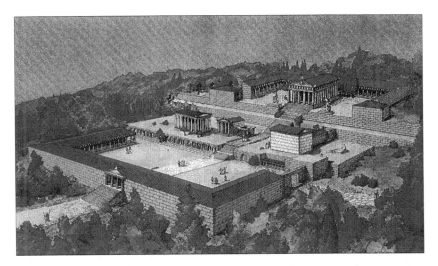

Reconstruction drawing of the Asklepieion.
From: M.S. Kiapokas, *Hippocrates of Cos and the Hippocratic Oath*.

My wife had just finished her residency in pediatrics, and I had completed mine in family medicine, both at the University of Colorado. We were in the early stages of a year-long around-the-world trip. A year off—after seven years of intense studies—to decompress and reconnect. We had an itinerary that included adventuring to twenty countries, immersing ourselves in different cultures, broadening our knowledge of history, connecting to ancient sacred sites, and doing medical volunteer work in the Ukraine and Nepal.

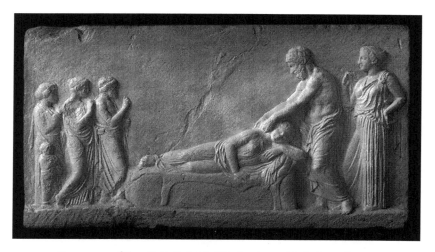

Fragment of Bas-Relief. A Girl Patient on a Bed, Aesculapius
Stands above Her. Credit: Wellcome Library, London.

Taking the interisland ferry from Rhodes to Kos was a choppy, nauseating hydrofoil ride. My wife could have fed the fish along the way, thanks to her motion sickness, but instead opted for the modern approach, using the sanitary bag under the seat. Luckily, I have never suffered from motion sickness and attribute this to a tolerance inherited from my maternal grandfather, a Navy Rear Admiral who fought in the Pacific during World War II and survived.

After my wife improved, I contemplated the mysteries of Kos. Arriving mid-day, we grabbed our backpacks and disembarked across the small plank, down the wooden pier of the small port. Theresa was still a bit green, but quickly rebooted once her feet felt solid ground. Hmm, hold off on the ouzo tonight, I decided. Looking over the sun-bleached map inside the tourist information hut, I could see that the island is relatively short—only twenty-five miles long—part of a Dodecanese mountain chain submerged underwater except for the protruding tops. Many tourists stop here en route to Turkey, a short ferry ride away.

Known today for its beautiful Aegean Sea beaches and temperate climate, it's been a hub for winemakers, medicine, and academia since at least 500 BC. After talking to the local guide at the ferry port, we checked into a family-run hotel. Tossing our packs on the bed, we didn't waste any time heading out to explore the town a bit, eventually stopping at the archeological museum.

The museum has a small collection of local Greek and Roman antiquities, including sculptures, pottery, and intricate mosaic tiles. After viewing a Hellenistic head of Hippocrates, I looked over at an elderly gentleman who was observing it with me.

What brings you to Kos? I asked—greeting him with a big smile. "I'm here for a reenactment of the Hippocratic Oath at the asclepieion tomorrow." *That sounds amazing*, I replied. *Are you a physician?* "Yes, from England. I'll be attending the ceremony with a large group of members of a medical history society. How about you?" he asked? *I'm in the early stages of a round-the-world trip with my wife. We're both physicians and finished our residencies this summer.* "That's great. Good for you guys," he said. "Being that you are both young physicians, I'd be happy to invite you along if interested." I hastened to reply, *That would be amazing!! Count us in!*

The next morning—along with thirty other physicians from around the world—we found ourselves in the ancient temple, immersed within minutes in beautiful flute music; then a procession of islanders draped in togas and wearing olive-wreath crowns proceeded to the central, open-air area, where we stood waiting. The priest guided us in reciting the Hippocratic Oath in unison.

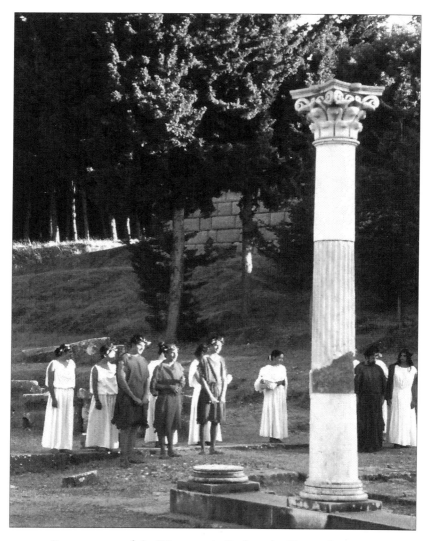

Reenactment of the Hippocratic Oath at the Kos Asclepieion
by locals for approximately thirty physicians from around
the world, including the author

As we stood in the scattered-stone remnants of the temple, sensing the sights and sounds, I noticed that something deep was happening simultaneously amongst us all. Reciting the oath felt timeless, creating a bond, an unusual flow of energy that I couldn't process at the time, as if something was being realigned. Standing at this site, I felt a tingle down my spine that would recur at many sacred sites to come. I was elated that both my wife and I had had the honor to attend, but knew there was deeper, perhaps synchronistic meaning to the fact that we happened to show up magically for this rare reenactment.

Reciting the oath made me reflect further on this legendary healer. All graduating medical students recite his oath, but know little of him beyond these words, along with and the image of a wise-appearing, bearded man cloaked in a toga.

What did the "Father of Medicine" believe and contribute to the early stages of medicine? Unfortunately, little is recorded of his life that can be verified. The Greeks regularly composed speeches and attributed them to famous people in the past; over time this gave rise to stories—such as that Hippocrates cured the great plague of Athens—that may or may not be true.[12] By legend but probably not reality, he lived to be over one hundred years old. By ancient, detailed, genealogy, he was—depending on which genealogy you follow—the seventeenth, eighteenth, or nineteenth male descendant of Asclepius himself.[13] Jouanna reminds us: "That the history may seem legendary to us is another matter. Aristocratic families, for their part, believed in the factual basis of their genealogies sufficiently to go to the trouble of engraving them in stone inscriptions that were meant to be read by everyone."[14]

This was a promising place for my wife and I, as young doctors in our twenties, to connect to the seemingly primal origins of modern medicine. These Asclepiads (descendants) were, in the strict sense of the word, hereditary noble families that, whether physicians or not, closely preserved the secrets of medicine—knowledge they passed orally from father to son down through the centuries.[15]

Even after Hippocrates moved to Thessaly, after his parents died and his children were adults, his protégés carried on his legacy.[16]

Here, at Kos, as mentioned, "the technique of healing differed from that at Epidaurus and elsewhere, where cures were effected by suggestion. At Kos, as is revealed by inscriptions, patients underwent treatment at the hands of physicians on lines laid down by Hippocrates."[17] We do know that Hippocrates thought disease developed from natural causes rather than being a punishment of the gods or having a superstitious cause.

Hippocrates appreciated the important spiritual and energetic relationship of the mind and body, while at the same time developing techniques to heal with herbal medicines and by surgical means when necessary.

Spyros G. Marketos, a historian at the Department of the History of Medicine, Athens University Medical School, records some of the current facts about his teaching:

> He was one of the most significant figures in the history of science because he separated the art of healing from the notion of demons, superstition and magic. Diseases had a logical interpretation, they were no more a curse of the gods or a punishment to man due to divine wrath. The Hippocratic diagnostic system, based on logical reasoning, observation and belief in the "healing power of Nature," formed the basis of medical practice. . . .

"For the physician," as it is written in one of his relevant works, "it is undoubtedly an important recommendation to be of good appearance and well-fed, since people take the view that those who do not know how to look after their own bodies are in no position to look after those of others. He must know how and when to be silent, and to live an ordered life, as this greatly enhances his reputation. His bearing must be that of an honest man, he must be towards all people honest, kindly and understanding. He must not act impulsively or hastily; he must look calm, serene and never cross."

The Hippocratic physician was basically both a craftsman and scientist, accompanied into his workshop by an audience of pupils and other bystanders, who discussed the diagnosis and treatment of every case. When he went to the patient's home he had the duty to persuade not only him but also the relatives. He followed the more communal character of life in antiquity, which did not permit any special discretion or intimacy in his behavior. If he made a reputation for himself, then this was publicized in other towns and he probably attracted patients from other regions or he was invited to visit other cities. . . .

The Hippocratic physician attended cases of every type, and did not refuse to do his best for a case because the use of an instrument was demanded. He was thus no specialist, but he combined traditional internal medicine with surgery.[18]

I often wonder how a conversation between Hippocrates and Leonardo da Vinci would have gone. Perhaps both were connected to the same timeless level of consciousness, making them infinite Renaissance beings.

The distinguished professor emeritus Vivian Nutton, of the University College London, is a preeminent authority on Greco-Roman medical research. He dived deep into early medical texts, including new finds in papyri and other documents, resulting, in 2004, in his *Ancient Medicine* (Sciences of Antiquity series), widely described as "the most comprehensive and up-to-date survey available." In the sixth century BC and the early fifth, he explains in the updated second edition, "the boundaries between magic and medicine were almost nonexistent." By 350 BC, however, the shaman-like healing that had been so prevalent was "marginalized."[19]

Historical accounts attest to amazing healings in Kos and at the numerous other asclepieia. One inscription in Epidaurus contains the testimony of Ambrosia:

> Ambrosia from Athens, blind in one eye, came here as supplicant to the god. Walking around the temple she made fun of some of the curing methods she saw, because she could not believe them. It seemed impossible to her that a paralyzed or blind person could be healed by a dream. Falling asleep she had the following dream: Like if the god himself stood by her telling her she would be healed. But he asked her to pay for the cure by dedicating to the temple a silver pig as a reminder of her disbelief. After saying

this, he ripped her eye and poured medicine into it.
In the morning, Ambrosia left the temple all healed.[20]

Due to widespread illiteracy, most records were oral. Written documents were copied by hand—and copied again. Nevertheless, from the scant supply that did not disappear, we know the following: Patients would begin by purifying themselves at a sacred spring, followed by offering a sacrifice. White-robed, they would then undergo, prior to entering the temple, a second purification. Spending the night, they would (if fortunate) receive a vision, in which the god or a sacred snake or dog cured their ailment. In other cases, a dream provided helpful information or a riddle that the patient relayed to temple physicians (priests) for interpretation.[21] Similarly, today, Jungian or Freudian dream analysis may be performed by psychologists to help detect underlying mind and body ailments. The modern-day process being more passive, in ancient times the patient was thought to be treated in a different dimension or realm during or after the dream.

Only remnants remain of the powerful asclepieion at Kos. Less than half the original marble walls and columns are standing. Not only did looters steal statues, but the Knights Hospitaller of Rhodes (the Knights of St. John) used a lot of the stone, as well as from other local historic sites like the agora, in the fifteenth century to build Kos Castle.[22] This is a familiar phenomenon— the classic example being the Rome Coliseum, which once had marble seats and siding. But over time, in addition to suffering earthquake damage, its marble and travertine (a marble-like stone) were looted, sold, or given away. Several sources, including prolific Giuseppe Lugli, professor of ancient Roman topography at the University of Rome (1933 to 1961), report that "in the year 1451–1452 alone, 2.522 cartloads were taken from the site to be used for buildings of the Vatican and for the walls of Rome."[23] Many Greek ruins suffered the same fate.

I wondered about the thousands of healers trained within asclepieion walls. Did they return to their villages to treat the sick or only treat within the temples? According to Nutton, the Hippocratic physician might work from home or travel to find patients.[24] How did they maintain the latest medical and spiritual knowledge to continue the best healing available at that time? After thousands of years, why did contemporary developed nations disregard the mind-body connection, as well as the importance of spirituality in healing? Surely, the great scientific innovations and breakthroughs by Kepler, Galileo, Newton, and others shifted our worldview towards science and technology, disconnecting us from the art of healing—and from the relationship to nature that was the precursor to our scientific mind set. In 1928, Sir Alexander Fleming discovered the first true antibiotic, penicillin, leading to the development of many other antibiotic classes in the 1940s to '60s. The fortunate but one-sided development of life-saving medications and surgical techniques diverted interest away from the mind-body healing techniques of the past.

But to take a step much further back, not so many centuries ago nature dominated the planet. It's hard to fathom, but in 1350 only about 370 million humans inhabited the globe.[25] With travel difficult (on foot, on horseback, on camel, by ship) and reading restricted to the literate minority, the worldview closely reflected home, where nature met the eye at every turn. As of early 2019, there are 7.7 billion people inhabiting our planet!

Following my experience on Kos, I often pondered how the spiritual training Hippocrates gave his physicians differed from that of modern medical schools. My estimate is that at least half their training was spiritually based.

My medical school and residency was mostly void of instruction to support patients spiritually, or psychosocially around the birth of a newborn, not to mention how to deal emotionally with the death and dying or suffering of a loved one. We had to learn that one on our own. I'm not saying I desired a minor in divinity or psychology or a shamanic apprenticeship, but simply a deeper understanding of the human psyche to help patients through major events.

More importantly, now that I've practiced medicine for over twenty years, I've discovered that to keep patients centered and healthy, it's equally consequential to manage small events and interactions over years. I am convinced a deeper understanding of the mind-body connection, our alignment to nature and the universe, and how we might integrate these concerns into more effective healing desperately needs to be reintroduced into our medical education. By and large, this has been long lost—with some exceptions—and is overdue for a rebirth into the halls of our medical schools and beyond. As the pendulum swings back in the opposite direction, books like *Happiness & Health: 9 Choices That Unlock the Powerful Connection between the Two Things We Want Most*, by Rick Foster, Greg Hicks, and Jen Seda, MD, one of the founders of the Mayo Clinic Complementary and Integrative Medicine program, remind us that positive thoughts, emotions, and actions affect our health.

The roots of many of today's medical practices can be traced back to the woeful, inefficient, non-standardized state of medicine in the U.S. in 1910. We lagged behind our European counterparts. To tackle the situation, Abraham Flexner and the (Johns) Hopkins Circle traveled around the country and analyzed models, such as medical education in the German universities, to produce their recommendations. According to "The Flexner Report—100 Years Later," published in the *Yale Journal of Biology and Medicine*, one third of American medical schools were "rated of such poor quality that closure was indicated. . . . A majority of the medical schools were rated as defective with low admission standards, poor laboratory facilities, and minimal exposure to clinical material. Medical education at the turn of the century was a for-profit enterprise that was producing a surplus of poorly trained physicians. The enactment of state licensing laws put teeth into the indictments of the report. Flexner sounded the death knell for the for-profit proprietary medical schools in America."

"The Flexner Report—100 Years Later" acknowledges the resulting reorganization of medical training was "awesome in the breadth and depth of understanding and discovery." Though successful in imposing a much-needed scientific basis of medicine, it produced dire consequences. Over the long haul it transformed medical education to what I experienced, as do most medical students today: a scientific, hyperrational approach, primarily devoid of the art of patient care.

A $14 million "SUPPORT study" ("The Legacy of SUPPORT," 1999) "found that more than 40 percent of families were unhappy with the fashion in which their loved ones were cared for as they died." In summary, "The Flexner Report—100 Years

Later" stated: "The profession appears to be losing its soul at the same time its body is clothed in a luminous garment of scientific knowledge."[26]

Assessing humankind, Carl Jung put it well: "Through scientific understanding, our world has become dehumanized. Man feels himself isolated in the cosmos. He no longer is involved in nature and has lost his emotional participation in natural events, which hitherto had a symbolic meaning for him . . . No river contains a spirit, no tree means a man's life. . . . His immediate connection with nature is gone forever, and the emotional energy it generated sunk into the unconscious."[27]

Our Native American tribes, including the Hopi, Lakota, Navajo, Maya, Aztec, and many others around the world, have maintained the connection with the cosmos, but in my opinion 90 percent of humans on this planet have not. That fact is one of the major reasons I wrote this book.

Our modern belief that science and technology can fix anything led us to embrace quick fixes through the "sick care model." These blinders deter us from the logical transition to a preventative, "stay well model." Many large institutions are adding wellness and integrative medicine into their marketing to appear well rounded, but none have integrated this program throughout their subspecialized niches. Why? There's more money to be had from a cardiologist stenting your blocked vessel than what a hospital-employed nutritionist and meditation instructor can bill for helping you naturally lower your cholesterol, decrease stress, and prevent the need for the stenting procedure.

Being in the front line of care as a family physician, I found it obvious that at least half our efforts should be towards preventative research, strategizing towards proactively enhancing the health of our community rather than reactively responding to acute or chronic disease.

Genomic research is focused primarily on identifying the cause of specific disease, cancer, or illness, but I'm hopeful to see researchers devote an equal amount of effort to finding ways to reduce inflammation and discover how to improve our longevity and quality of life. What I will call preventative genomics.

This noble quest to stomp out disease lacks balance and—without inquiry into preventative markers—will fall short. Why not identify early in life those of us at risk for cancer, depression, or neurologic conditions such as multiple sclerosis, then research ways to dramatically reduce this risk? Will taking extra Vitamin D reduce our risk for multiple sclerosis, as suggested by preliminary studies at Oxford University, New Jersey Medical School, and the Maastricht University in Holland,[28] or can we only see that those of us with higher Vitamin D are at lower risk, since no one wants to fund further research that won't make money? Looking similarly for genes that put us at risk for developing Alzheimer's and Parkinson's and then researching ways to reduce that risk by decreasing neural inflammation is just one example of an early preventative genomic approach. Discovering which genes make Native Americans more at risk for diabetes than other ethnicities may help in targeted dietary therapies.

Simply imagine tending to your garden. Just pulling the weeds will not guarantee the growth of healthy veggies. They need appropriate light, water, and nourishment. Similarly, to stay well, we must search for ways to nurture our healthy DNA, just as in our gardens we want to prevent the expression (growth) of unhealthy, weed-like genes. Imagining our body as a thriving garden that is well tended to, perhaps we will achieve more optimal health. We don't want to default to a weed killer.

The multinational agrochemical biotech corporation Monsanto—whose name is being retired, in a recent acquisition by Bayer—has claimed a central position in the world of genetically modified seeds, or "organisms" (GMOs), and its proprietary chemicals. What could be wrong with plant technology—emphasizing "plant breeding," including "gene editing"—that creates insect-and-weather resistance?

For one thing, plants developed resistance to the chemical that was supposed to kill them: "To date, glyphosate resistance has been confirmed in 24 weed species worldwide, including 14 in North America (Heap 2012). Glyphosate-resistant weed populations have been confirmed in 29 states and two Canadian provinces."[29] Another drawback is below.

Not so well known is the fact that gene giants have, through navigation of intellectual property laws, used them "to commodify the world seed supply."[30] An unhealthy root structure is a byproduct. By contractually making farmers use *their* pesticides and seeds, the giant has in many cases destroyed American and international farms. A Reuters news report in 2011 warns that, "Repeated use of the chemical glyphosate, the key ingredient in [Monsanto's] Roundup herbicide, impacts the root structure of plants, and 15 years of research indicates that the chemical could be causing fungal root disease, said Bob Kremer, a microbiologist with the US Department of Agriculture's Research Service."[31]

In August 2018, a trial, the first of its kind, resulted in a $289 million jury verdict—now under appeal—against Monsanto on the charge that over thirty years it intentionally concealed that glyphosate-based Roundup is "probably carcinogenic to humans"—and was therefore liable for non-Hodgkin's lymphoma of a former school groundskeeper. "Monsanto still insists it is 'safe.'" Top U.S. retailers continue to carry the product, but the filing of lawsuits has jumped into the thousands.[32]

The conclusion I draw is that apparently Monsanto, which once contracted with the U.S. government to manufacture agent orange to spray over Vietnam, would rather have farmers use their chemical herbicides and GMO seed than develop cheap, non-GMO seeds and support natural, effective ways of managing a less-productive but certainly more sustainable and healthier field.[33]

The 2018 merger with Bayer is only adding concern, according to a survey: "Nearly 1,000 farmers in 48 states, representing all sectors of farming, were asked about the pending merger and more than 935 expressed concern, with top worries being increased pressure to practice chemical-dependent farming and reduced choice for purchasing seeds and other inputs."[34] Just as corporate greed has dominated agriculture and energy, we are also dominated by Big Pharma. Physicians get reimbursed for a short visit to prescribe a depressed patient an antidepressant, but poorly reimbursed for counseling. The same goes for weight-loss counseling to prevent or treat Type 2 diabetes. Guidelines for treatment of depression, diabetes, and many other conditions are overseen and written by physicians and others with financial ties to drug companies.

For a decade, I was a volunteer on a medical-guideline committee, representing the Colorado Academy of Family Physicians. Together, based on available research, I and physicians from various subspecialties developed the best local guidelines and recommendations for colon cancer screening, high blood pressure treatment, and many other conditions. What I noticed while reviewing national depression guidelines was concerning, however. Many of the physicians who had written the depression guidelines in other states and nationally were receiving huge speaker fees from drug companies to discuss the latest antidepressants. How could these guidelines not have extreme bias? Rather than looking at the bigger picture of treating the patient more holistically, there was a focus on drug-based therapy.

The *Journal of the American Medical Association* (*JAMA*) retrospective study looking at antidepressants concluded that while substantially beneficial in cases of severe depression, the benefits of medication over placebo "may be minimal or nonexistent, on average, in patients with mild or moderate symptoms." Yet the national depression guidelines would make physicians and patients think that Prozac and other SSRI (selective serotonin reuptake inhibitor) antidepressants were a panacea, making everyone happy. I couldn't believe the blatant bias before my eyes and saw similar biases showing up in other guidelines, often by physicians who had received speaking-engagement payments from drug companies listed in the disclosures.[35]

The majority of medical research today is funded by drug companies; every clinical medical journal is half full of pharmaceutical ads. Not to mention the direct-to-consumer advertising on television. We must scrutinize the rationale of these corporate entities that are promoting their lucrative products.

Preventative genomics can reintegrate the wisdom of the ancients and re-explore the benefits of spirituality and mindfulness as we observe favorable changes in our DNA. Neuroimaging brain mapping—such as by fMRI (which measures changes in brain blood flow) and QEEG (which records and analyzes the brain's electrical activity, its brainwaves)—is already showing beneficial results from mindfulness-based therapies. Again, we must be willing to do research beyond the profits of drug-based interventions and invasive procedures, and trust results conducted with the highest level of scientific vigor. Bringing mindfulness, nutrition, and lifestyle therapies back on line will provide a balanced, more effective prevention-and-treatment strategy. Without this we will fail as we continue to battle rising rates in diabetes, suicides, multidrug-resistant bacteria, and cancer. Our 17 percent-of-GDP healthcare expenditure in the United States far exceeds that of other developed countries, yet our overall health falls far behind. Why? We are putting too much emphasis on profit-making drugs and procedures, rather than preventative strategies that promote stress reduction and healthier lifestyles. We need our medical system, when possible, to emphasize therapies that get to the root cause of conditions such as Type 2 diabetes.

Hippocrates and other ancient practitioners were truly patient focused—unlikely afflicted by for-profit entities and the bureaucracy that today's healthcare providers encounter. They taught and practiced medicine in a pure, unbiased manner without the influence of drug reps, hospital CEOs, or insurance companies making decisions on life-saving medications or procedures. Today the direct-to consumer drug and hospital advertising is making the situation even worse.

The collapse of these ancient civilizations—from the Greeks to the Egyptians, Maya, and others—led to a loss of thousands of years of medical wisdom. Decreased interest in ancient medicine was further eroded by the promises of science and technology, antibiotics, and cold surgical steel.

Why did these advanced civilizations go under? According to UCLA scientist Jared Diamond—in his Pulitzer Prize-winning book—over the last thirteen thousand years the fate of societies was often dependent on "Guns, Germs and Steel." The subtitle is *A Short History of Everybody for the Last 13,000 Years.* Diamond's argument is persuasive:

> The book's title [*Guns, Germs, and Steel*] is a reference to the means by which farm-based societies conquered populations of other areas and maintained dominance, despite sometimes being vastly outnumbered—superior weapons provided immediate military superiority (guns); Eurasian diseases weakened and reduced local populations, who had no immunity, making it easier to maintain control over them (germs); and durable means of transport (steel) enabled imperialism. . . .

Diamond argues that Eurasian civilization is not so much a product of ingenuity, but of opportunity and necessity. That is, civilization is not created out of superior intelligence, but is the result of a chain of developments, each made possible by certain pre-conditions.[36]

While I agree with Jared Diamond, I feel the demise of these advanced cultures resulted from the impact of three things: Power, Greed, and Disrespect for others. The possession of weapons further accelerated their demise or other civilizations' demise. Disease and starvation played a lesser role. The decimation of Native Americans was due to the impact of Europeans with guns and to the germs they spread. Leaders' (and a culture's) ego grew as their empires expanded and superior weapons were developed to further overtake or subdue others. A thirst for more and more permeated the consciousness, eventually leading to greater immoral acts of greed, as demonstrated by the Roman pillaging and conquering of peaceful societies. Put simply, once the yin/yang balance of masculine/feminine energy is moderately disrupted locally or globally by the leaders and/or the populace, decline begins. We are witnessing that severe imbalance in our country today.

Locally we are witnessing how the entrenchment of U.S. gun owners has resulted in the refusal to ban assault weapons and large-capacity ammunition magazines often used in high-profile mass murders. As our world leaders continue to fail to curb the growth of nuclear arsenals, we could find ourselves perilously close to global catastrophe. President Trump recently, in 2019, pulled out of the 1986 Intermediate-Range Nuclear Forces Treaty. This will potentially accelerate the arms race, just as his pulling out of the Paris Agreement jeopardizes success in combatting climate change. We can only hope a more comprehensive, modernized arms treaty is negotiated (with adequate verification), bringing in China. In regard to the Paris Agreement, thankfully, "city, state, business, and civic leaders across the country and around the world are ramping up efforts to drive the clean energy advances needed to meet the goals of the accord and put the brakes on dangerous climate change—with or without the Trump administration."[37]

Likewise, there is a yin/yang balance in medicine. We've lost that. Ancient medicine, such as systematic acupuncture (about 2,000 years old), has this yin/yang balance. We would do well to bring back the best of our ancestors and cautiously avoid being arrogant in thinking that modern medicine is the only solution, just as we need to further embrace renewable energy and permaculture, and not the petroleum and agrochemical industry. Integrating these traditions in a balanced, open-minded way will help us regain optimal health to shift our genome more naturally and favorably.

Our goal should be to artfully integrate East/West, Ancient/Modern medicine to achieve this optimal yin/yang, masculine/feminine balance for best outcomes and not high profits. We cannot let corporate interests force the latest pill or procedure on us rather than simply changing our diet in many cases. I am not condemning all medications, but feel that we need to use them appropriately, after natural therapies have been tried without success or need to be augmented. For example, being told you need weight loss by a medication followed by gastric bypass is bad medicine unless you've worked very proactively with a nutritionist to try a ketogenic-diet and exercise routine. Typically, an inadequate trial with less-proven diets is performed, thus favoring the surgical option. This is also true in the joint-replacement (knees and hips) industry, where many could benefit from nonsurgical management, including weight loss and regenerative stem-cell therapy.

Darwin was correct in his field observations of the adaptive transformation of the beaks of evolving finches in the Galapagos archipelago and Cocos island. But he didn't realize that we can modify ourselves here and now, *and not just over generations and hundreds of years.* A favorable environment, and not just a popularized Darwinian "survival of the fittest" by competition, can change your DNA for the better.

The purpose of this book is to challenge the reader and our scientific community to explore and embrace the benefits of spirituality and mindfulness to our DNA. It's about being neuroplastic and looking to concepts beyond the conventional—paddling down the lesser-known rivers, those not explored by well-known, rock-starlike spiritual authors. My goal is to help bring into the twenty-first century the lost teachings from the asclepieion and our great ancient-medicine forefathers. This exploration will provide insight on how to rekindle spirituality and mindfulness to improve your health, quality of life, and longevity by *turning on* the good things in your DNA! Every chapter in this book relates to how to enhance your DNA. Let's begin the journey . . .

Chapter 2

Shift Your DNA for Wellness and Longevity with Mindfulness and Meditation

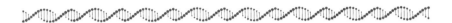

My discovery of the benefits of mindfulness began as I pursued my passion in preventative medicine. I felt the best strategy to do this was on the front lines of patient care in family medicine. Only there could I interact with all ages, making the biggest impact. The trail was much more of a challenging adventure than anticipated.

After graduating from residency in family medicine in '96 and doing a year of international travel and medical volunteer work, I set out on my career at a large Kaiser Permanente clinic in Denver. Prior to this position, the last patient I'd seen was in a remote rural village in the Langtang mountains of Nepal. As they filed in one by one over a week my wife and I saw several hundred patients in a small stone hut with nothing but a wooden table, chair, crude exam table, stethoscope, notepad, and basic medical supplies.

Leaving that primal hut of human suffering and entering this beautiful modern clinic was a bit of a culture shock! Below me was a pharmacy, an optometry clinic, and a lab, and on the second floor adjacent to my office were several other doctors, including family physicians like myself, pediatricians, and obstetricians. Reflecting on the previous year's journey, I smiled as I looked out through the large windows from the upper floor across the atrium to panoramic mountain views of the front-range, wondering deeply what lay ahead. Would I make this my long-term medical home, or was it a small side excursion on the trail? Hustling from room to room, I and my fellow physicians each greeted our patients in pressed, logoed white jackets, with barcoded nametags and stethoscopes, feeling like super docs stamping out disease! But were we?

We were lauded for seeing twenty to twenty-five patients a day, returning ten to fifteen patient phone calls over lunch, and then staying in the office till 8 p.m., finishing up our notes in the new electronic medical record. Exhausted, with additional labs and patient questions to answer, we would eventually call it a day and head home. It didn't take long to realize I was on a hamster wheel, spending the majority of my time writing prescriptions and working to meet productivity quotas of the corporate supervisors. Everyone was to be treated by an evidence-based guideline, using formulary medications, referral processes, etc., within a very limited amount of time per patient. Those that sought to do a longer interview, diving deeper into the patient's condition, or who contemplated integrative therapies would either fall behind or potentially get called out for recommending something not mainstream. Suggesting acupuncture for lower-back pain might elicit the rebuke: *Why would you do that, when you could just prescribe ibuprofen or Percocet? Why would you recommend meditation for someone with anxiety? There's Xanax for that.*

We were advised to type, code, and complete our notes while seeing the patients, which distracted us—removing eye contact except for an occasional glance away from the computer screen. We were not "present" for the patient, but "present" for the computer, documentation, and coding. I laughed as a so-called "super-user physician" of the electronic medical record coached a group of us over lunch about how we could position the screen at an angle, smile, and glance at the patient in a more personal manner. Seemed as phony as a politician trying to gain my vote with a smile and wave.

I refused to put that wall up, so I'd type in the basics and do my best to listen and look in their eyes rather than succumbing to a dehumanizing, robotic appointment accompanied by a fake smile as I typed. A ten-minute visit left all of us writing a quick Rx, reaching for the door handle, and moving onto the next. It didn't take long before we felt the stress of this structure impairing our art of healing, leaving many of us burnt out and patients feeling disconnected. Technology and corporate management had found a way to destroy the doctor-patient relationship, placing us on a spreadsheet rather than allowing us to be effective healers.

Sure, quick appointments worked well for simple things like strep throat and urinary tract infections, but not for my patients struggling with depression or chronic inflammatory conditions, stress-related conditions, and autoimmune disease. Besides, most came in with a list of three or more major issues or conditions, not just one.

After two years on a hamster wheel, feeling remorse over not being able to do the deeper work for my patients, I was asked to join the faculty at the University of Colorado to teach residents. I left.

This was much more enjoyable, but with the clinic pressured by issues of managed care, we were likewise forced to see more and more patients to keep the doors open. Teaching opportunities were constrained, and patient care visits shortened. During this time I expanded my studies and exploration in integrative and holistic medicine, and in teaching the Integrative Medicine elective for residents, I brought in acupuncturists, energy medicine workers, meditation instructors, nutritionists, and others so the med students could learn about therapies beyond the ScriptPad and scalpel.

Many have asked: why didn't you want to become a famous heart surgeon like your father? The simple answer has always been that I desire to keep my patients' hearts healthy through diet, nutrition, and lifestyle rather than cracking their chest and replumbing their arteries. The majority of surgical interventions, whether for coronary artery bypass, joint replacement, skin cancer, etc., are preventable. Trauma, genetic predisposition, and age-related disease account for the rest, which are typically not preventable unless one forgets to buckle up or wear a helmet in high-risk sports. It's concerning that over 210,000 patients die undergoing surgery each year in the United States.[38] Complications from surgery, such as postoperative infection, stroke, and blood clots, are not to be ignored either.

After five years of academia I decided to open a private practice. This was a scary jump, to leave a salaried position with benefits and go at it alone. I had never imagined I would encounter so much dysfunction in medicine that it would lead me to have to create my own practice. I went to countless meetings on healthcare reform and even volunteered on a diverse physician panel to contribute ideas to Senator Ted Kennedy in DC. Few of our recommendations made it into President Obama's Affordable Care Act. The majority of the plan was dictated by for-profit managed care. Regardless of the rapids and canoe-wrapping boulders along my medical journey, I found my practice growing well; it was successful in a year. I was able to develop the work of my dreams— emphasizing prevention, wellness, and integrative, functional, and regenerative medicine. What I call simply good medicine.

Instead of seeing sick patients all day, I found myself much happier helping the majority stay well.

I began to understand my patients' concerns more comprehensively by switching to longer visits, some lasting up to ninety minutes. I could flow with their thoughts and feel intuitively into their physical, mental, or spiritual imbalances. I also made time to meditate most days, instead of running myself to the ground as I had in the other settings. I dove into the latest research in the human genome, studying epigenetics and nutrigenomics. Epigenetics evaluates the global effect of lifestyle, nutrition, and environment as it *turns on or off* particular genes. Nutrigenomics is the narrower focus on how foods affect our genes in a positive or negative way—the greatest potential benefit coming from cancer and other disease prevention

My practice quickly transitioned, so that the majority of visits were aimed at optimizing wellness. To assess how individuals were aging, I began performing telomere testing. Stress and smoking, for example, can shorten telomeres, which are end caps protecting our DNA. I was an early adopter of genomic screening, way before 23andme.com, and continue to utilize it when patients are interested in risk stratifying themselves confidentially for various cancers, Alzheimer's, mental health disease, diabetes, autoimmune, methylation disorders, and more. Of course, the limitations and pitfalls of genetic testing are discussed up front, and we review the results, to take advantage, where possible, of any opportunity to prevent the manifestation of disease.

Mainstream medicine does a reasonable job in prevention, primarily through vaccines and cancer and cardiovascular screening. Of course, I still embrace and recommend these strategies. But a greater emphasis should be placed on "primary prevention" in all settings. The wall we encounter is that insurance rarely covers counseling for weight loss, smoking cessation, mental health, and mindfulness-based coaching.

An example of primary (proactive) prevention would be advising someone to lower cholesterol early on with diet and exercise, rather than having that person be rushed to the hospital for a chest pain, getting a stent in a heart vessel, and thus then in secondary prevention (reactively) putting the sick person on a diet and medication to lower his/her cholesterol *after* the injury to prevent *another* heart attack down the road.

In my judgment, the most important primary preventative strategy may be mindfulness—whether it prevents you from having heart disease or from hurting yourself or another in being overstressed. It may be the best violence-prevention strategy for our nation and world too, which desperately needs an intervention to reduce hate crimes such as mass shootings. In *The Biology of Belief: Unleashing the Power of Consciousness, Matter and Miracles*, stem-cell biologist Bruce Lipton eloquently discusses, with supportive research, how positive thoughts and beliefs can express

DNA that's beneficial to your health, and conversely if they are negative: "Our positive and negative beliefs not only impact our health but also every aspect of our life. . . . While we cannot readily change the codes of our genetic blueprints, we can change our minds and in the process, switch the blueprints used to express our genetic potential. You can live a life of fear or live a life of love. But I can tell you if you choose a life of love, your body will respond by growing in health."[39] In addition to the benefits positive beliefs have on your personal genome, new studies are shedding light on how meditation and mindfulness can positively affect your DNA.

In 2009 Elizabeth Helen Blackburn, a Tasmanian-born molecular biologist and biochemist, was awarded, along with Carol W. Greider and Jack W. Szostak, the Nobel Prize in Physiology or Medicine for discovering the importance of telomeres and an enzyme called telomerase in protecting our chromosomes.

Telomeres, those protective DNA sequences that act like end caps to our chromosomes, shorten as our cells divide. Just as most things fray with wear, so do the protective telomere DNA caps at the ends of your chromosomes. Having this cap as a buffer helps prevent genetic defects of lost information as the cell divides. The enzyme *telomerase* helps keep those caps intact. Research tells us we can enhance our telomerase activity through stress reduction, healthy diet, exercise, and other strategies. Enhancing or maintaining optimal telomerase activity improves the telomere length, thus, the life span of a cell, and thus your lifespan as well.

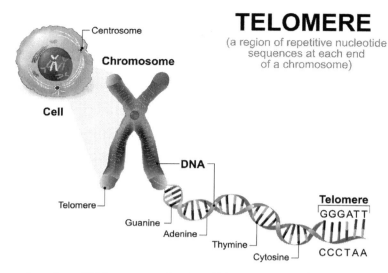

TELOMERE

(a region of repetitive nucleotide sequences at each end of a chromosome)

Location of Telomeres on the tips of chromosomes (Shutterstock)

Looking into this model, researchers at UC San Francisco, in an analysis published in 2009, wrote: "Telomere length has now been linked to chronic stress exposure and depression. This raises the question of mechanism: How might cellular aging be modulated by psychological functioning? We consider two psychological processes or states that are in opposition to one another—threat cognition and mindfulness—and their effects on cellular aging. . . . We propose that some forms of meditation may have salutary effects on telomere length by reducing cognitive stress and stress arousal and increasing positive states of mind and hormonal factors that may promote telomere maintenance."[40]

In 2011, a UC Davis Center for Mind and Brain study reached a similar conclusion about participants attending a three-month meditation retreat. They determined that the emphasis on mindfulness and purpose of life led to increased perceived control, and decreased neuroticism, "with implications for telomere length and immune cell longevity."[41]

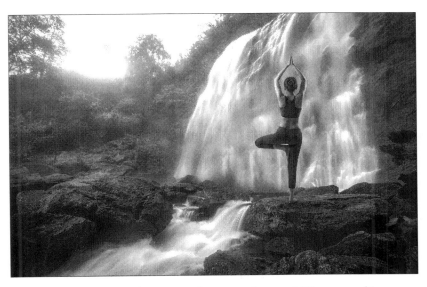

Enhance your telomeres with yoga and nature! (Shutterstock)

Another case study, published in *The Journal of Alternative and Complementary Medicine* in 2015, demonstrated improvement in telomere length and reduction in blood cortisol (stress hormone) levels and inflammatory markers (Interleukin-6) with yoga.[42] Additionally, the growing field of psychoneuroimmunology continues to show how stress adversely decreases the effectiveness of the system's ability to fight infections and the growth of malignant tumors.

Can one prevent or treat cancer through mindfulness and stress reduction? I feel it's possible—yes. But it will be extremely difficult to prove, as it requires funding and a randomized controlled-study design. Let me be clear. I'm not saying that those with cancer should ever forego therapy recommended by an oncologist, but that mindfulness as an adjunct could potentially improve your odds of successful treatment.

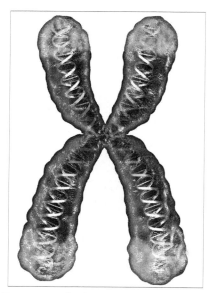

Depiction of telomeres on tips of DNA
(Shutterstock)

There are billions of Big Pharma dollars going into immunologic-based cancer drug therapies. But we will be lucky to find even a million to further study the effects of meditation or mindfulness on cancer prevention and complementary treatment, since it can't be patented and made profitable on Wall Street. Regardless, there is enough existing evidence, in my opinion, to support mindfulness-based activities (in addition to exercise and a healthy diet) in cancer reduction. For example, to assess whether parachutes work or not, we don't have a randomized controlled trial. Imagine being randomized to drop out of a plane without a parachute packed. Similarly, commonsensical therapies can be useful, especially if there's no potential harm. Just don't meditate under a palm tree with large coconuts!

In 2016, a Zen meditation study demonstrated this positive effect by showing longer median telomere length in expert meditators compared to nonmeditators. An emphasis on acceptance and compassion is pertinent to Zen meditation. Prior studies, by Q. Conklin et al. (2015) and N. A. Schutte and J. M. Malouff (2014), also associated mindfulness-based practices with longer telomeres. From these studies, it can be concluded that all types of meditation can help improve your telomere length.

Conklin et al., in their 2015 article, even found that telomere length can be improved in as short a time as a three-week meditation retreat. The authors concluded, "This finding suggests that the contemplative, behavioral, and environmental shifts that accompany participation in a full-time, residential, and silent meditation retreat may lengthen leukocyte telomeres—perhaps by facilitating the participant's cultivation of adaptive mental qualities, which mitigate psychological stress and counter stress-related telomere shortening."[43]

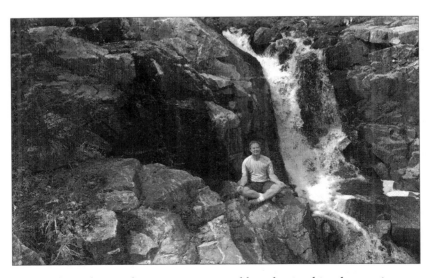

The author meditating in nature and lengthening his telomeres!
Photo by Jonette Crowley

One can deduce that individuals who manage stress well, and pursue mindfulness-based activities will have longer telomeres, promoting greater longevity and overall health. By contrast, being under high levels of stress may shorten telomeres, potentially increasing the risk for a myriad of health problems, including depression, anxiety, obesity, diabetes, heart disease, Alzheimer's, colds, and gastrointestinal conditions, to name a few.

Elissa S. Epel and Elizabeth H. Blackburn, et al., demonstrated accelerated shortening of telomeres related to stress in 2004.[44]

In a 2006 *Annals of Neurology* study, telomere length was noted to predict an increased risk of death after stroke as well as risk for cognitive decline and dementia.[45]

A 2009 study showed that short telomere length increased the risk of death by cardiovascular disease in men. Perhaps the hostility component of the type A personality plays a role.

Do shortened telomeres cause cancer? We haven't found the evidence yet, but they are notedly shorter in patients with cancer, diabetes, high stress, and heart disease. As mentioned, with shorter telomeres, the risk of death is higher in patients recovering from major events such as heart attack and stroke. A recent meta-review of the evidence thus far, undertaken by Masood A. Shammas and the Dana Farber Cancer Institute (Harvard Medical School), points out:

> Telomeres therefore play a vital role in preserving the information in our genome. As a normal cellular process, a small portion of telomeric DNA is lost with each cell division. When telomere length reaches a

critical limit, the cell undergoes senescence and/or apoptosis. Telomere length may therefore serve as a biological clock to determine the lifespan of a cell and an organism. Certain agents associated with specific lifestyles may expedite telomere shortening by inducing damage to DNA in general or more specifically at telomeres and may therefore affect health and lifespan of an individual. In this review we highlight the lifestyle factors that may adversely affect health and lifespan of an individual by accelerating telomere shortening and also those that can potentially protect telomeres and health of an individual.[46]

Similar research on a Parkinson's-disease test case in 2016 by Ada G. Marsh, Matthew T. Cottrell, and Morton F. Goldman joins in the chorus of scientists lining up behind this same cutting-edge outlook to recognize that "epigenetic modifications of genomes [play] central interacting roles in genetic determinants of health and disease." This Marsh, Cottrel, Goldman research adds that gene activation is not likely to occur in the presence of methylation (for a definition of that, see below). Significantly, "This gene expression regulation directed by epigenetics in a large part explains why an individual is *not simply a pre-programed reflection of a parentally inherited genome*, but instead during their life they can develop alternative paths toward different outcomes of health and wellness."[47]

In species ranging from rodents to humans, this shift in DNA makeup *based upon environment* has been demonstrated to occur rapidly. Recently, NASA studied the genomic shifts in astronaut Scott Kelley (in space for a year), compared to his identical twin, Mark, living on Earth. Seven percent of the change in his genome has remained in the two years since, so that the twins are no longer identical genetically. The weightless environment and perhaps high levels of radiation in the space station likely influenced methylation in Scott.[48]

What is methylation? Here's a very easy-to-understand definition from my friend, the author of *The Thyroid Cure*, Michelle Corey:

> Methylation is the latest buzzword in the health industry, and for good reason. It's a biochemical process involved in almost all of your body's functions! What is methylation? Without getting too technical, think of billions of little on/off switches inside your body that control everything from your stress response and how your body makes energy from food, to your brain chemistry and detoxification. That's methylation and demethylation.[49]

Looking beyond the telomere caps for our chromosomes, ongoing research is shedding light on how lifestyle, diet, and mindfulness more deeply affect our DNA.

Through this epigenetic process, bad genes can be expressed (turned on) during stress, or with mindfulness-based activities and relaxation they can be repressed (turned off). Stress raises inflammatory markers in the blood and reduces immune function, while alternatively, mindfulness and less stress will express genes that reduce the inflammatory markers and aid in healing and regeneration. Mindfulness, as expected, can also enhance immune function.

A 2016 systematic review of twenty randomized controlled studies, compromising 1,600 participants and meeting rigorous inclusion criteria, was undertaken by a team from the University of Southern California. Authors, Black and Slavich summarized the benefits in three categories below:

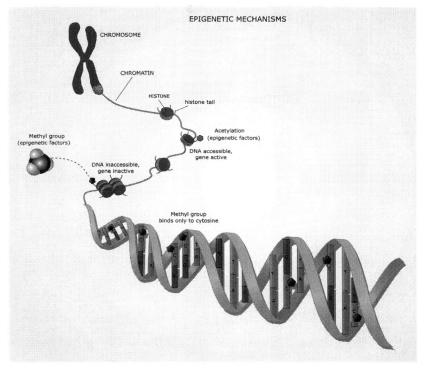

Epigenetics and the Methylation Process (Shutterstock)

Reduced inflammation via

- decreased NF-kB transcription activity (which reduces the number of copies made of this inflammatory DNA sequence)

- decreased CRP levels (a global marker for inflammation in your body)

Increased cell-mediated immunity via

- higher CD4 + T-cell count/activity (this is what drops in HIV patients and leads to infections.)

Slowed biological aging via

- increased Telomerase activity (see prior discussion on telomerase)

The authors conclude that "mindfulness meditation appears to be associated with reductions in proinflammatory processes, increases in cell-mediated defense parameters, and increases in enzyme activity that guards against cell aging."[50] They emphasize that further studies are needed and that for greater benefit, mindfulness should be a sustained daily practice. As with exercise and diet, it can't just happen at a retreat or spa weekend, but should be maintained throughout the work week and beyond.

I love retreats, but see them as building on my foundation at home. It's just like climbing mountains on the weekend for me. I have to maintain a level of fitness that allows me to have a "peak experience" and a higher likelihood of reaching the summit, just as a meditation retreat will take me deeper inside or into the stars if I've done the work upfront.

Interestingly, the majority of expensive but effective immunotherapy drugs for psoriasis we see in television ads address many of the same pathways as mindfulness. Researching in 2018, I found the average annual cost for medications like Humira, Tremfya, Enbrel, and Xeljanz is about $50,000. Good luck with insurance covering any of it these days! Personally, I'd rather do ten island meditation retreats and improve my daily routine for far less than fifty grand. If mindfulness, stress reduction, and an anti-inflammatory diet and supplements are ineffective, then consider adding in low doses of these medications if needed. Remember, there are many side effects beyond the pocketbook.

In addition to reducing stress through mindfulness, an often more important process is to learn how to release negative and/or traumatic experiences. Since this can be a root cause of acute and chronic stress, failing to address and deeply release deep-seated negative experiences can limit the benefits of therapies. Meditating or praying to a place of forgiveness and compassion for oneself or others can often release painful experiences, but for many they can't go there or access it. Particularly those who witnessed a murder, were raped, or experienced other horrific crimes.

Veterans and others suffering from moderate to severe PTSD (Post-traumatic Stress Disorder) all too often spiral into severe depression, then suicide, regardless of psychotherapy and medications. According to the U.S. Veterans Administration, effective strategies include psychotherapy (various forms of talk therapy) and antidepressants. Clearly this isn't enough, since roughly eighteen to twenty-two veterans commit suicide daily.[51]

While I am not a trauma therapist, I have seen many patients find success with integrative therapies, including EMDR (Eye Movement Desensitization and Reprocessing), acupuncture, neurofeedback, and Rolfing, to name a few. Of all those I've witnessed, the most powerful therapies have been Holotropic Breathwork, plant medicine, MDMA (3,4-Methylenedioxy methamphetamine), and facilitated psychotherapy.

Though MDMA-facilitated therapy and plant medicine are not legal in the U.S., I'm hopeful that with ongoing research they will re-emerge as an approved therapy. I'll discuss these therapies more in Chapter 8. Breathwork should be offered by the VA and other large institutions for those who need to clear traumas that can't be mitigated by psychotherapy.

What is breathwork? Breathwork can be as simple as "take a deep breath" when someone cuts you off in traffic, to more advanced forms, including the following:

- Pranayama yogic breathwork, such as Ujjayi, Dirga, Sitali, Bhramari, Kapalbhati, Nadhi Shodhan, Kumbhaka, Lion's breath, and more

- Kundalini Breath of Fire (shallow, rapid breathing)

- Holotropic Breathwork by the Grofs (hyperventilation and non-ordinary states) and Breath Mastery (Dan Brulé)

- Conscious Breathwork, radiance, shamanic, integrative, transformative, Vivation, and many more

By far, the most powerful breathwork I've experienced is the Holotropic type, developed by Czech-born psychiatrist Stanislav Grof and his late wife, Christina, and birthed from a long lineage, including "consciousness research, anthropology, various depth psychologies, transpersonal psychology, Eastern spiritual practices, and mystical traditions of the world."[52] This method creates a non-ordinary state of consciousness. As explained in their book *Holotropic Breathwork: A New Approach to Self-Exploration and Therapy*, this method forges much deeper than psychotherapy, providing just what our overstressed and disconnected society needs. While embracing Jungian theories and building on experiences from over thirty years, including psychedelic therapies, they've assisted individuals to clear deeper wounds and traumas, channeling them to their higher self.

Gurpreet Kaur Gill, a Colorado friend and facilitator of Conscious Breathwork—another powerful form, like Holotropic—has witnessed amazing breakthroughs. Talking with me one afternoon, she shared a few memorable examples that continue to fuel her passion as a facilitator: some clients had been having suicidal ideations; others were caught in a web of manipulation and abuse; others were depressed, feeling anxious, lost, and unsure of life, from all walks, and socioeconomic slices of life.

One Type A powerhouse of a businesswoman—who on all accounts was leading a very successful life—had experienced immense trauma, PTSD, and negative body association (in the form of multiple rapes, including one while drugged and unconscious; a mom disassociated from the moment of her birth; to a dysfunctional on-again off-again relationship, and more). She arrived in Gurpreet's practice in a delicate state, barely holding it together. After a series of breathwork sessions, where there were multiple breakthroughs, including allowing herself to feel tender emotions and cry rather than constantly leaning into her warrior self and "pushing through it," she finally feels safe in her body despite all she has lived through; able to love and to embrace her feminine self; recognizing the immense power to heal, to be whole, that lives within her own body and its intelligence. To this day, she credits her multiple breathwork sessions as assisting her to truly love herself despite all the negative life experiences and in helping to solidify her connection to the Greater in her day-to-day life.

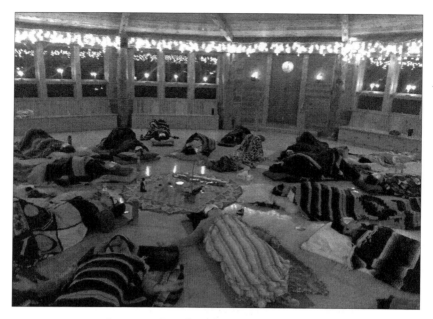

**Conscious breathwork session facilitated by
Gurpreet at Starhouse near Boulder**

Another client, in his first session, shared that he had been crying daily for the last six months—one reason was known (a romance breakup); others were not readily accessible. He was immensely desperate for a shift. Truly, within one single session, he birthed himself anew—clearing what had been holding him stagnant and breathing fresh life-force energy into his being. He laughed, saying, "Breathwork shifted my paradigm in one session, where fifteen years of talk therapy weren't able to." For some, a single session truly is the equivalent of a decade of therapy—and admittedly, there is a time and place for talk therapy, but for him, breathwork was the time to get to the root of what was ready to shift and/or be cleared.

He reflected that breathwork had permitted him "to feel the full power of ME," of the immense power living within his own being, rather than relying on others to reflect or to affirm his abilities to him. He continued to work with Gurpreet; three sessions later, he was well on his way to living his version of his best life—the once-daily tears replaced with an immense zest for life, adventure, and service.

Finally, Gurpreet shared the story of a young soul sexually manipulated and abused by her partner, a leader of a cult-like group. Disassociated from her body on many levels, she dove into her first session—a group session, nonetheless. Her body shook, moving of its own accord during the breathwork as it unwound trauma, tears, and screams of release. Finally, a loud and powerful, "NO!" ripped out and reverberated through the space. That was her initial breakthrough moment—reclaiming of self, her body, her being, and her voice. She has had several more sessions since—all immense in their unfolding. To see her today, a shining, beaming, radiant young woman, you would never guess her history. She has returned to living her life, going to school and pursuing her dream to herself become a breathwork facilitator.

Facilitators like Stanislav, Christina, and Gurpreet gently guide participants to experience expanded states of consciousness, higher states of oneness, and compassion, and to infuse a greater since of responsibility for our planet and its inhabitants. In my opinion, this type of breathwork or working with plant medicine (as discussed in Chapter 8) offers the deepest clearing of negative energies, while connecting us to the light of the universe.

In summary, start by dipping your feet in the pool through meditation. Once you experience the multitude of benefits emerging from the expression of healthy DNA, dive deeper if needed. A deeper dive into non-ordinary/expanded states with the help of a therapist or shaman can help you cleanse and release old traumas, making you feel elated like a Labrador Retriever shaking himself off after a swim in the lake.

Chapter 3

Resonating to the Sacred Geometry of Art and Architecture

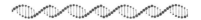

One spring afternoon after a busy morning of seeing patients, I walked over to a local restaurant, just a couple hundred feet from my office. I'm a regular there, grabbing lunch at least twice weekly, and have gotten to know most servers. I go there for my usual mahi-mahi fish tacos, coleslaw, iced tea—and the fresh air on the outdoor patio.

On this day a new waitress showed up at my table with a Flower of Life tattoo on her forearm. I'd seen plenty of sacred geometry elements tattooed and incorporated into owls, snakes, dragons, birds, fish, and beyond, but this was a simple, pure Flower of Life. Attending meditations and shamanic gatherings in Boulder, just north of my home, has exposed me to much more body art than the average physician, but this basic representation quickly caught my attention. In my office, I had just hung a commissioned oil painting of this form the week prior.

Trying not to be flirty, I said, "Hey, nice Flower of Life!" She smiled back, thanking me, and I asked, "What does it mean for you?" She said, "Ya know, I just feel connected to the geometry of it." Intrigued, I remarked, "There's more to it than meets the eye." She returned a smile, and I intuitively knew she was on the path to understanding it more. The Flower of Life is composed of overlapping circles evenly spaced to form a symmetrical hexagon; this sixfold base is arguably the geometric foundation for the creation of life; I'll unpack this thought below. We find this pattern in numerous other connections in nature and the universe.

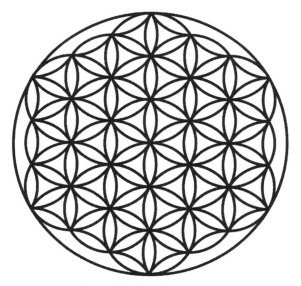

Flower of Life (Shutterstock)

Global interest in sacred geometry has grown exponentially over the last decade, but in ancient times sacred geometry was appreciated and applied in temples and artwork, as it has its origins in nature. The number of books, courses, and emerging art in this genre attests to its popularity today. Whether it is a phenomenon of individuals relating to it through spiritual growth, love of nature, art, architecture, authors, or other factors, it is refreshing to observe.

Its contributions to civilization began thousands of years ago with the Egyptians, Indians, Greeks, Romans, Chinese, Inca, and others. Most fascinating is how sacred geometry in architecture and art follows nature in symmetry, proportion, and mathematical principles. According to Robert Lawlor, the author of *Sacred Geometry: Philosophy & Practice*, "the starting point of ancient geometric thought is not a network of definitions or abstractions, but instead a meditation on a metaphysical Unity, followed by an attempt to symbolize visually and to contemplate the pure, formal order which spring forth from the incomprehensible Oneness."[53]

Many of the early contributions were birthed in the southernmost tip of Italy by Pythagoras of Samos (c. 570–500 BC), a close contemporary of Buddha. His Pythagorean theorem enriched sacred geometry, as did his discovery of the intervals of harmonic ratios, including the golden ratio, and the healing nature of music. Not to mention that his Pythagorean triangles segued to the later discovery of the Fibonacci sequence. In view of his genius, he is often considered the father of music, as well as of philosophy, and the major founder of the Essene Movement (Jewish Pythagoreans). I will expand on harmonics, cymatics (sound geometry) and sound healing more in Chapter 5.

The Pythagorean theorem, still taught in school, states that in a right triangle, "the square of the hypotenuse (the side opposite the right angle) is equal to the sum of the squares of the other two sides."[54] In the next chapter, I will go into detail about the golden ratio and the Fibonacci sequence.

On a spiritual level, his open-minded integration of spirituality and our physical world gave him and other intellectuals, including contemporary, much greater insight than if limited to our tangible 3-D world.

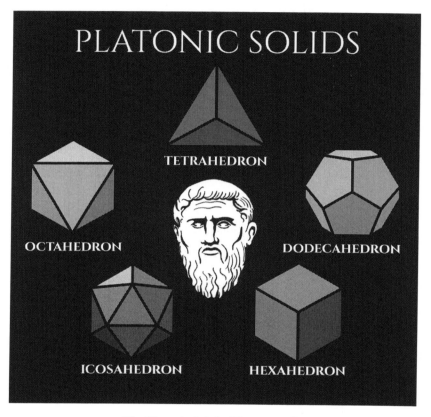

The Platonic Solids (Shutterstock)

Well over a century later in Athens, Plato, a critical philosopher, was one of the earliest to bring geometry to the masses. Greek historian Plutarch summarized: "Plato said God geometrizes continually."[55] Plato considered geometry and number the ideal philosophical language.[56] In his book *Timaeus* he deliberates on the four basic elements of the world proposed before him by Empedocles: earth, air, fire, and water. Though Plato mentions aether by name, it is left to his most famous student, Aristotle, to add it as a fifth element (in order to include the celestial bodies), though not by name; later commentators called the fifth element aether. The five platonic shapes that traditionally align to these elements are the cube (earth), tetrahedron (fire), octahedron (air), icosahedron (water), and dodecahedron (aether). Aether was considered in ancient times to be the material that filled the space of the universe.

The platonic solids, described by Plato c. 350 BC, were probably discovered a thousand years earlier than Plato, by Neolithic man. Stones found in Scotland dated to the Late Neolithic period (approximately 3000 BC) are in the Ashmolean Museum at Oxford.

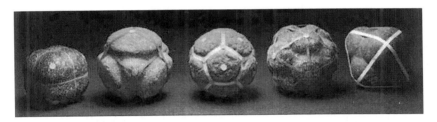

Five-thousand-year-old Scottish stones likely representing the earliest known forms of the platonic solids.

In *Time Stands Still: New Light on Megalithic Science*, Keith Critchlow, Professor Emeritus at the Prince's School of Traditional Arts in London and a former professor of Islamic Art at the Royal College of Art, postulates that Neolithic man used these "cosmic volumes" (five platonic solids) to help align Stonehenge and other great circles in Britain. He went on, "What we have are objects clearly indicative of a degree of mathematical ability so far denied to Neolithic man by any archeologist or mathematical historian." Some archeologists dispute the claim that the stones represent a full set of the platonic solids, citing a questionable icosahedron, and further state that the balls are simply art, and have nothing to do with math. I disagree, however, and am sure that great artists and thinkers such as Da Vinci would quickly see both the mathematical and artistic elements equally.

Following the Greeks, the Romans integrated this geometry into their art and architecture too. Vitruvius, the Roman architect and military and civil engineer (born 80–70 BC, died sometime after 15 AD), promoted it conceptually in the first century BC in his book *De architectura*. He states, "Architects, taking their lead from nature, designed the tiers of seats in theatres on the basis of their investigations into the rising of the voice, and tried, with the help of the mathematician's principles and musical theory, to devise ways in which any voice uttered onstage would arrive more clearly and pleasantly at the ears of the spectators."[57] He believed the ideal architect, being both theoretical and practical, needed a comprehensive understanding of mathematics, nature, geometry, astronomy, astrology, and science to design practical, aesthetic, and spiritual architectural plans. To summarize, he felt buildings should be *firmitas, utilitas, venustas*—solid, useful, and beautiful.

Vitruvius incorporated this sophisticated geometry into many public buildings and temples. Centuries later, around 1490, Leonardo da Vinci, while apprenticed in Andrea del Verrocchio's workshop in Florence, used some of Vitruvius's initial sketches of the human body to draw the final Vitruvian man.

In this drawing, *Vitruvian Man*, or *The proportions of the human body according to Vitruvius*, Leonardo famously inscribed the human body inside a circle and square, demonstrating two fundamental geometric patterns of the cosmic order. Later works by him such as the *Mona Lisa* also incorporated divine order. We even find the Flower of Life in Codex Atlanticus, a twelve-volume collection of his sketches and writings.

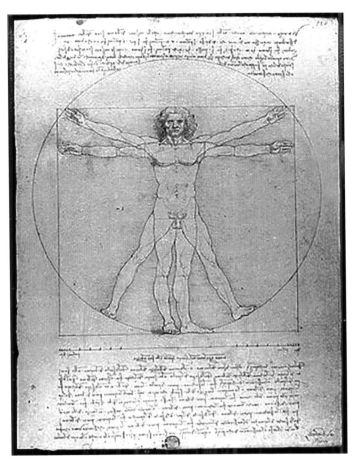

Vitruvian Man **by Leonardo da Vinci, c. 1487 (iStock)**

Sacred geometry has played a major role in the art and cosmology of most religions. In *Sacred Geometry*, Robert Lawlor popularized a passage from *The Mathematics of the Cosmic Mind: A Study in Symbolism*, by Theosophist L. Gordon Plummer. Plummer noted that "the Hindu tradition associates the icosahedron with the Purusha. Purusha is the seed-image of Brahma, the supreme creator himself, and as such this image is the map or plan of the universe."[58]

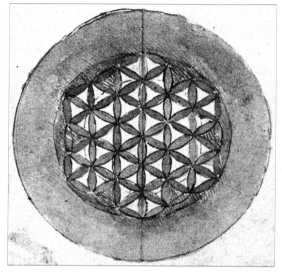

One of Leonardo's drawings (between 1478 and 1519) of what is now called the Flower of Life), Codex Atlanticus fol. 309v

Others have hypothesized the universe to have dodecahedral (a twelve-sided polygon) geometry. In 2003 in *Nature*, French and U.S. cosmologists tackled a scientific conundrum regarding temperature at different scales in the oldest light in the universe—the microwave-radiation sky. To solve the thorny problem, they postulated that the universe is shaped like a dodecahedron; contrary to being infinite, filled with dark matter, they wrote, it is "a simple geometrical model of a finite space—the Poincaré dodecahedral space."[59]

Many people, including some cosmologists, have for some time felt that the universe itself is fractal.[60] I particularly like a quotation from a pioneering scientist, Nassim Haramein, the Director of Research for Resonance Science Foundation: "Everything in the universe emerges from an underlying unified organizational field patterning and gives rise to the self-similar scalar fractal organization of all living systems."

Fractalization occurs when irregular or fragmented patterns repeat themselves so as to be self-similar as they go to different scales, from large to smaller forms or vice-versa. Also known as "expanding symmetry." As American astrophysicist Margaret Geller said, "One of the great challenges of modern cosmology is to discover what the geometry of the universe really is." On a cellular level, the internationally famed pioneering scientist Bruce H. Lipton states, "Mathematical studies have found that fractal geometry is the best way to get the most surface area (membrane) within a three-dimensional space (cell).[61] Why does it matter to us? I believe that appreciating fractal and sacred geometry aligns us with the healing energy of the universe. Furthermore, we can gain greater insights into universal consciousness and further activate, or epigenetically shift, our DNA. The geometry of the universe is believed to be contained within the Flower of Life. So regardless of whether the universe is a dodecahedron, icosahedron, tetrahedron, or the newly proposed amplituhedron, the core elements are derived from Flower of Life.

Also nesting in the Flower of Life, in addition to the platonic solids, we find the "Metatron's Cube." It becomes visible when we connect the center point of each of the thirteen circles in the Flower of Life. Metatron is an archangel.

Developmentally, the mammalian embryo has the "seed of life" geometry during the early blastocyst stage. The "seed of life" is also nested within the Flower of Life.

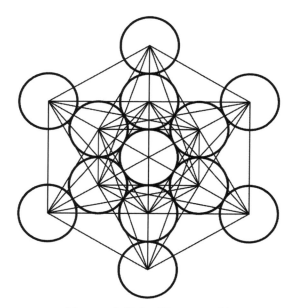

Metatron's Cube (Shutterstock)

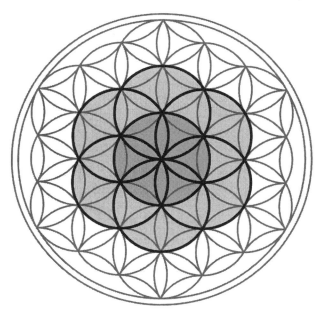

The seed of life (shaded) within
the Flower of Life (Shutterstock)

One can hypothesize that, amazingly, the genesis of the Earth's elements, humans, and the universe are in accord with the geometry of the Flower of Life.

From an ancient archeological standpoint it is an enigma that the engraved Flower of Life geometry at the Osiris temple in Abydos, Egypt, is also found in the temples in the Forbidden City (China) and in Japan; ancient synagogues in Israel; the Golden Temple in Amritsar, India; the city of Ephesus, Greece; the great mosque-cathedral "the Mezquita" in Cordoba, Spain; and thirteenth-century Italian art—not to mention the work of alchemists—to name a few.[62] As it's beyond the scope of this book to go further into this topic, for readers who want to more comprehensively understand the depth and meaning of the Flower of Life, please read Drunvalo Melchizedek's *The Ancient Secret of the Flower of Life,* volumes one and two.

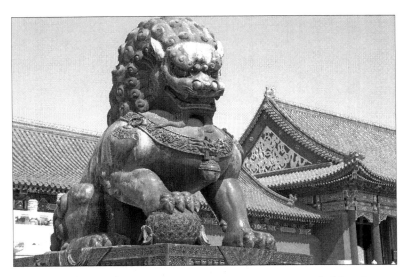

Flower of Life Sphere under "Guardian Lion" paw, Forbidden City (Shutterstock)

From an experiential standpoint, my fascination with architectural sacred geometry began during a month-long college elective to London in 1985. We went there to study the history, art, and architecture of London and southern England through the teaching of a history and philosophy professor who accompanied our group of fifteen. After exploring the historic sites of London, we ventured out to the countryside to Salisbury and Stonehenge. Firing up my Sony Walkman and some '80s rock, I peered through my window seat as our small bus bumped through the pastoral landscape.

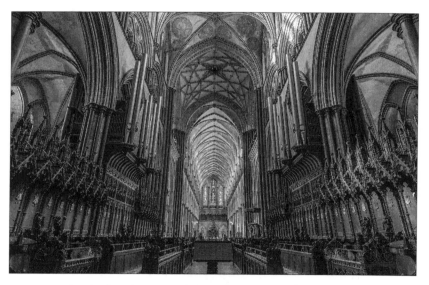

Vaulted Ceilings at Salisbury Cathedral (Shutterstock)

Already in the parking lot, we could see the massive buttresses of the 750-year-old medieval Salisbury cathedral, with its impressive spire rising 404 feet into the blue sky. The spire is the tallest in all England. Just as tall rainforest trees have large buttresses to support their height and vertical weight, the engineers, with their stonemasons, applied this natural adaptive feature to keep the cathedral walls from bulging out, imploding under the weight. Entering on the south side, we stared down the narrow naves and up at the geometry of the ribbed vaulting high above us. Gazing up at the interlaced, arched ceiling, I felt a sense of awe, in part due to intuiting a geometrical connection to God and Spirit.

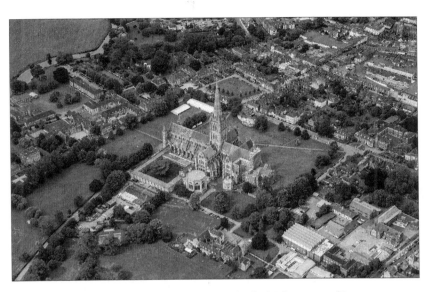

Aerial View of Salisbury Cathedral (Shutterstock)

As I was lost in contact with the space, our professor lectured. Not sure if I retained much of that! We were near the center of the Cross-pattern floor plan. He walked us over to a column, pointing to where you could see it bowing slightly inwards from the sheer weight of the upper structure. While he delved into the construction, I was enchanted by the expansive elements—the curves, angles, and ratios so magically integrated into this majestic site.

Interestingly, the cathedral may, as reported below in a 2014 news account, lie along a ley line that connects with Stonehenge:

> Another significant Wiltshire ley runs through Stone-
> henge, Old Sarum, Salisbury Cathedral and [the Iron
> Age hill fort] Clearbury Ring. Dowser Romy Wyeth,
> from Codford near Warminster, demonstrated to the
> BBC how a line of energy can be detected at the
> centre of Stonehenge, again at Old Sarum and run-
> ning through to the Cathedral Close and beyond.
> The subject of ley lines—at least what they repre-
> sent—is a controversial area, but the strength of evi-
> dence is compelling.[63]

A ley line is a hypothetical line that connects geographical, spiritual, or mystical sites. According to this theory, the lines connecting these sites create a field of energy, similar to a defined meridian
line used by Chinese acupuncturists to balance or heal the human
energy field. Others believe that a ley line connects Angkor Wat
to the pyramids of Egypt and Stonehenge. Hiking the Inca trail
years ago, I learned that the Incas had also created energetic lines,
using apachetas. Apachetas are similar to large cairns or stone
markers you might see while hiking to the summit of a mountain.
They used these like nodal points to connect the energy of Machu
Picchu and other sacred sites to the Inca capital, Cusco, which
they considered the naval of Pachamama (Mother Earth).

Seeing Salisbury Cathedral or any sacred site in a book had always intrigued me, but standing almost directly under the central
point of this three-dimensional structure, I felt more: a coherence
with it. Perhaps its alignment with a ley line amplified the sensation even more.

After Salisbury we journeyed to the nearby prehistoric site of Stonehenge. Shifting back in time 5,000 years, from a more cubic structure of the cathedral to this circular one, was an interesting sensation.

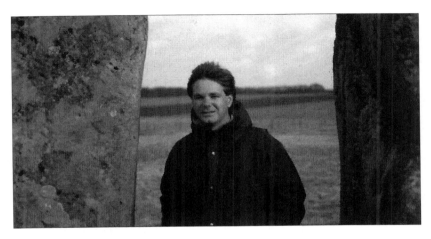

The author at Stonehenge, 1985

Back in the '80s we could walk around the circle, unrestrained by today's fence. Fascinated, I imagined ceremonies amidst its sandstones (Sarsen stones) weighing fifty thousand pounds and bluestones weighing up to eight thousand. According to English Heritage, in charge of caring for more than four hundred buildings and sites, the earliest here, a henge monument (that is, built in "a roughly circular or oval-shaped flat area enclosed and delimited by a boundary earthwork—usually a ditch with an external bank"),[64] was constructed around 5,000 years ago. "The unique stone circle was erected in the late Neolithic period about 2500 BC."[65]

In February 2019, the latest findings (reported in *Antiquity* magazine) detected that two particular Welsh quarries— Carn Goedog and Craig Rhos-y-felin—had bluestones removed c. 3000 B.C., coinciding with the start of the construction of Stonehenge. "Evidence suggests that workers used wedges to loosen pillars from the rock face and tied ropes to control their descent onto an artificial platform. Then, they may have laid timbers on top of the platform so they could be lowered onto a wooden sledge and hauled away."[66] The plot thickens. The article adds: "Collectively, this research conclusively invalidates the misconception that Pliocene or Pleistocene glaciers may have transported the bluestones to Salisbury Plain." The authors state:

> Almost 100 years ago, the geologist H.H. Thomas speculated that the bluestones had initially been incorporated into a "venerated stone circle" somewhere in Preseli, before making their momentous journey to Salisbury Plain. Around the same time, surveyors from the Royal Commission on Ancient and Historical Monuments (RCAHM) in Wales (1925) recorded the presence of a partial stone circle at Waun Mawn, perched above the source of a tributary of the River Nevern. This is located just 3km west of Carn Goedog and Craig Rhos-y-felin, 2km north-west of Cerrigmarchogion and 3km north-east of Banc Du. Yet no one—either at the time or subsequently—has investigated whether Waun Maun might be this former stone circle—potentially the original Stonehenge.[67]

Contemplating how workers transported these stones from 180 miles away, some weighing close to eight thousand pounds, was mind-boggling. According to Freddy Silva, best-selling author and researcher of ancient systems of knowledge,

Russian scientists monitoring EEG brainwave patterns inside the nave of Chartres discovered that the building's special harmonics have a noticeable affect [*sic*] on peoples' states of awareness. When combined with Gregorian chant—the kind of music these churches were designed to amplify—brainwaves go up [far] above [a] normal waking state.

At Stonehenge, the relatively simple series of rings and horseshoes that make up the world's most famous stone circle belie the fact that the positioning of the stones is governed by a complex geometric blueprint. In fact, it may be the only temple in the world that incorporates multiple sacred geometries: triangular, square, pentagonal, hexagonal, and heptagonal.[68]

Another thing I learned recently is that what I saw at Stonehenge did not survive intact like that. There were restorations. Here is a firsthand witness of when the reconstruction started:

Lady Antrobus observed the restorations at Stonehenge carried out in September 1901, resulting in an article she authored being published in the Saturday October 19th, 1901 edition of *Country Life*, in which she observed:

"The most dangerous and intricate piece of work to be undertaken was the raising to an upright position of the great monolith called the Leaning Stone, the king of the mystic circle and the largest in England, Cleopatra's needle excepted. This stone was one of the uprights of the great trilithon which stood behind the Altar Stone, and the Duke of Buckingham is said to have caused its fall by his digging and researches in 1620. The fallen upright is broken in two pieces and its lintel lies, as it fell, across the Altar stone.'"[69]

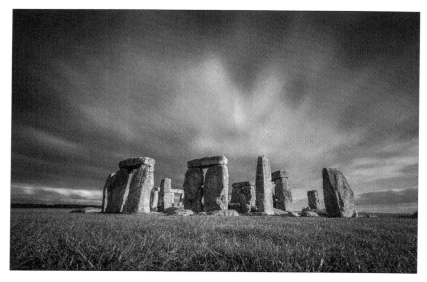

The powerful Stonehenge Circle (Shutterstock)

However, today's technology allows us to see much more perceptively when looking back in time, going not just above ground but underground. In my opinion, Stonehenge isn't a primitive structure, but a complex archeo-astronomic, spiritual structure whose ancient code and function won't be cracked until astronomers, archeologists, and present-day druids have a free-flowing forum of shared knowledge. Unfortunately, just as we see with medical research, archeologists and their institutions (universities, museums, etc.) prefer to function more within their professional box, limiting the potential for connecting the dots between astronomy, spirituality, and archeology. I'm hopeful to see a lot of collaborative work in all disciplines and institutions, moving forward in a win-win spirit.

Making a three-dimensional map of Stonehenge through underground surveys by instruments scanning three metres deep, "with unprecedented resolution," is revealing the site as much larger and more complex than initially perceived. The BBC News reported in 2014:

> Nishad Karim, a researcher at the University of Leicester, has used similar instrumentation to reconstruct 16th century Tudor tombs.
>
> She told the BBC: "Using GPR and other techniques, these researchers have been able to virtually see through the ground and explore what civilization looked like thousands of years ago."[70]

Among those leading the way at Stonehenge is fifty-six-year-old archeologist Vince Gaffney, who deployed various geophysical and remote-sensing techniques to discover buried elements. In "What Lies beneath Stonehenge?" (the *Smithsonian Magazine*), Ed Caesar writes, "Faint as the Avenue was, Vince Gaffney hustled along as if it were illuminated by runway lights." One of his notable discoveries, he describes as a

> "bloody huge" pit about five yards in diameter at the eastern end of the Cursus . . . much too large for a practical use—for instance, burying trash—because of the labor involved in digging it. In the archaeologists' minds it could only have ritual implications, as

> "a marker of some kind," Gaffney said. What's more, if you drew a straight line between the pit and the heelstone at Stonehenge, it ran directly along the final section of the Avenue, on the path of the sunrise on the summer solstice.
>
> "We thought, That's a bit of a coincidence!" Gaffney recalled. "That was the point at which we thought, What's at the other end? And there's another pit! Two pits, marking the midsummer sunrise and the midsummer solstice, set within a monument that's meant to be something to do with the passage of the sun."[71]

According to a 2016 publication of the Stonehenge and Avebury World Heritage Site Research Framework, some of the stones align with the solstices, so this was most likely a ceremonial worship site.[72] Multiple sources elaborate: "This Stonehenge monument—built in 3000 to 2000 BC—shows how carefully our ancestors watched the sun. Astronomical observations such as these surely controlled human activities such as the mating of animals, the sowing of crops and the metering of winter reserves between harvests."[73]

The alignment and the stone size and type were clearly critical to the designers, or they wouldn't have gone to such an enormous effort. Further research will likely show intricate geometric alignment with the stars, which may have assisted priests in achieving a more enlightened state during ceremony. Unfortunately, these geometries and alignments are not typically found in religious worship sites today.

Ptolemy's geocentric model from the second century AD standardized for over a thousand years that the predominant model of the universe had the Earth at the center; this meant the planets, the moon, the stars, and the sun revolved around the Earth. Today, we all recognize that we orbit the sun (heliocentric). Perhaps as we realize what a miniscule drop in the ocean our planet is and we are, we will align egos, churches, temples to the universe around us and ourselves. In my opinion, the universe has a multidimensional intelligence, and it's waiting for us to evolve and see the bigger picture.

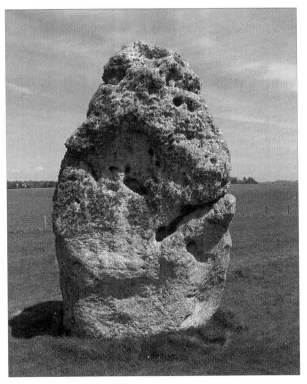

Stonehenge Heel Stone. Photo by Heikki Immonen

Let's move to Germany. In 1991, onlookers flying above Pömmelte spotted a henge, or "circular prehistoric monument constructed with wood or stone structures." This is now called the German Stonehenge:

> The henge has several concentric circles, the largest
> of which is about 380 feet (115 meters) across. . . .

> Ancient people built and used the henge-like monu-
> ment during the transition from the late Neolithic to
> the early Bronze Age, from about 2300 B.C. until 2050
> B.C., when it was destroyed—likely ritualistically.[74]

In the Dacian Romania capital of Sarmizegetusa, there was a large mountaintop defensive area with a sacred section called Sarmizegetusa (or Sarmisegetusa) Regia that now bears the title "the Romanian Stonehenge." Mighty warriors, the Dacians fought off the Roman invasion till early in the first century AD, as depicted famously in Trajan's Column, with its 155 carved scenes, in Rome. Difficult to reach, the capital began being studied by archaeologists only in the last century. As the UNESCO World Heritage website explains, "Built in the 1st centuries B.C. and A.D. under Dacian rule, these fortresses show an unusual fusion of military and religious architectural techniques and concepts from the classical world and the late European Iron Age. The six defensive works, the nucleus of the Dacian Kingdom, were conquered by the Romans at the beginning of the 2nd century [106] A.D.; their extensive and well-preserved remains stand in spectacular natural surroundings and give a dramatic picture of a vigorous and innovative civilization."[75] Here is a description:

> A number of rectangular temples were located there,
> the bases of their supporting columns still visible in
> regular arrays. Perhaps the most enigmatic construc-
> tion at the site, however, is the large circular sanctuary.
> This comprised a "D"-shaped setting of timber posts

surrounded by a timber circle, which was surrounded in turn by a low stone kerb. The original timber posts have long since rotted away, and the ones currently visible on the site are modern reconstructions in the original postholes. They help the modern visitor visualize the layout of the original construction, although the heights of the posts is completely speculative.[76]

This site is ideal for a discipline called archaeo-astronomy, which perhaps many of us have never heard of. But it exists, and simply involves analyzing the remnants of cultures to see what role the sky played in them. Sometimes researchers have to turn back the clock on the night sky to see the alignments that existed contemporaneous with when the circles, pyramids, and even the Sphinx were built and in active use. One researcher writes, with a flourish, that the Dacians were "perfect astronomers"; my source says, "amazingly precise":

> Very few know that the Dacians were [amazingly precise] astronomers, just like the Celts in northern England. At Sarmizegetusa there was a Dacian calendar, perhaps not as grandiose and popular as the [one at] Stonehenge, but more accurate.
>
> To be able to build such a calendar, the Dacians had to have extensive knowledge of mathematics, geometry, and astronomy.
>
> Like the ancient Egyptians, the Dacians studied and measured the stars. But unlike the pyramid builders, [they] used hourly coordinates, not horizontal coordinates as the Egyptians did."[77]

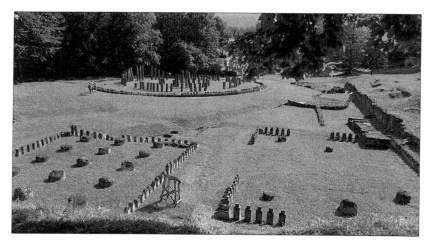

Sarmizegetusa Regia. Photo by Cosmin Stefanescu. "Sacred Zone" with circle, sundial, and additional celestial markers.

Back to my trip to Salisbury and Stonehenge in the '80s. Visiting Notre Dame de Paris later that month, I was mesmerized by the light penetrating the kaleidoscopic north-transept rose window. This style window has its origin in the Roman oculus (rounded central opening), that you can see in the famous dome of the Pantheon.[78] (See image.) To me, the multicolored, radiating rose-petal array inside the oculus broadcast oneness. Similar to what I feel, looking up at a dome of stars on a clear winter night in the mountains. I remember how, spellbound by the window, I momentarily experienced a portal-like sensation, feeling myself swept beyond the walls of this iconic sanctuary into a meditative state—just as if I were gazing deeply at a Buddhist mandala. The balance of the sharp, angular geometry of the vaulted ceilings and the soft, feminine curves of the ocular window and arches created a harmony that most people can drop into if they disconnect from the surrounding tourist chatter.

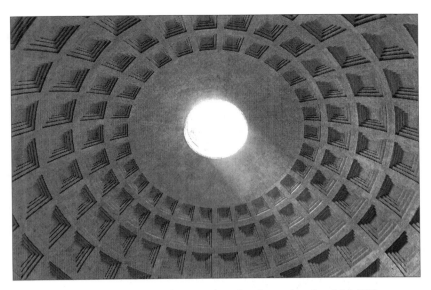

Pantheon in Rome with central oculus (completed c. 126 AD).
Photo by Wynand van Poortyliet on Unsplash.

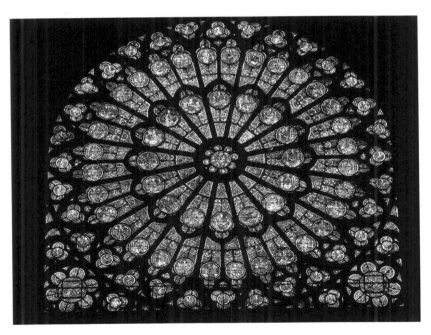

Notre Dame Rose Window (Shutterstock)

Soon one of my classmates nudged me out of trance and on to the next highlight. We climbed up the narrow stairs to the upper balcony near the bell towers. I was reminded of scenes of the hunchback of Notre Dame wandering along the narrow passageways in the old black-and-white movie, as we looked out over Paris and the Seine River. Pulling out my trusty Pentax SLR, I captured several black-and-white shots of the weathered gargoyles before heading back down the worn stones of the spiral stairs.

What inspired these architects to design sacred structures with such precise geometry and proportion? Were their concepts passed down from the ancients? How did the Freemasons obtain this knowledge? How did they find such skilled architects, craftsmen, the master stonemasons and glass workers—the laborers—and tools to construct with such precision and beauty? Is the intent to assist us in resonating with God or a higher spiritual state through a visual entrainment of our cortex? Visual brainwave entrainment can occur when we shift, for example, from one predominant brainwave pattern such as beta to alpha. In a research or clinical setting, strobing LED lights flashing at a specific frequency can induce these shifts. Perhaps the architects of certain cathedrals and temples were—knowingly or unknowingly—entraining us to higher spiritual states. Coupling that with the acoustics of choral music or chants and the resonance of a powerful pipe organ further amplifies these effects!

Research is needed to explore this hypothesis. As early as the 1940s a neuroscientist, Gray Walter, used a strobe (bright flashing light) to demonstrate these shifts in brainwave patterns through the cortex of the human brain. Long prior to this, around 200 AD, the Alexandrian mathematician, astronomer, geographer Ptolemy created colorful visual images by spinning a spoked wheel between the observer and the sun. Participants in Walter's experiments reported a sense of euphoria following the experience.[79]

Since then, numerous modern devices have been developed, including the PandoraStar, which I use in my practice. This unique LED-light therapy device emits varied frequencies of light from a Merkaba pattern (two triangles forming a six-pointed star) to induce different brainwave states aimed at promoting deep meditation.[80]

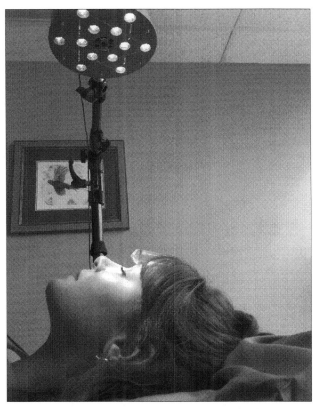

PandoraStar with Merkaba pattern in the
author's medical office, assisting a patient in deep
meditation while mantra music is playing through
the sound table she's lying on.

Inducing a gamma brainwave state with this photic (light-based) entrancement may, moreover, reduce brain inflammation and potentially be a treatment for early Alzheimer's. Dr. Li-Huei Tsai, of the Tsai Lab at MIT, found that in mice a flickering light at 40 hz/gamma frequency diminished amyloid plaque by 50 percent! As reported in "Unique Visual Stimulation May be New Treatment for Alzheimer's," Tsai says it's a big if. "But if humans behave similarly to mice in response to this treatment, I would say the potential is just enormous. . . . The bottom line is, enhancing gamma oscillations in the brain can do at least two things to reduce amyloid load. One is to reduce beta amyloid production from neurons. And second is to enhance the clearance of amyloids by microglia," Tsai says.[81]

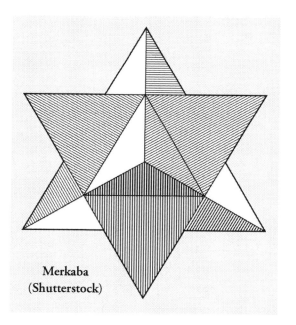

Merkaba
(Shutterstock)

The Merkaba is discussed in mystical traditions, such as the Kabbalah. I will come back to it later; it is widely described, in an energetic sense, as a vehicle of interdimensional travel.

Exploring southern Spain one fall, I headed off to Granada to see the Alhambra palace, where I was expecting a *traditional* Moorish site. But pleasantly surprised, instead I found flowing water integrated into sacred geometry. Sites that integrate water in a sophisticated way have always felt more balanced and activating to me and attuned to nature. Standing tall on a hill overlooking the town of Granada, the Alhambra palace complex offers a delightful exploration into Moorish architecture; it was originally built, in 889 AD, as a small fortress; later, in the fourteenth century, the Moorish emir Mohammed ben Al-Ahmar, of the emirate of Granada, built a palace on top of the remains.[82] During this time it was ruled by Arabs and Berbers.

After climbing the hill and entering the grounds, I walked into the courtyard of the fourteenth-century Palace of Lions.

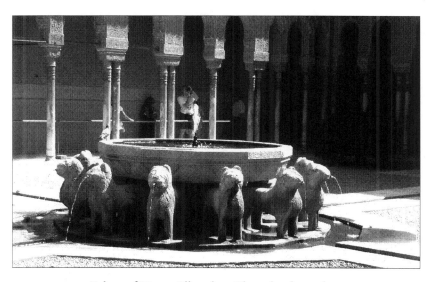

Palace of Lions, Alhambra. Photo by the author.

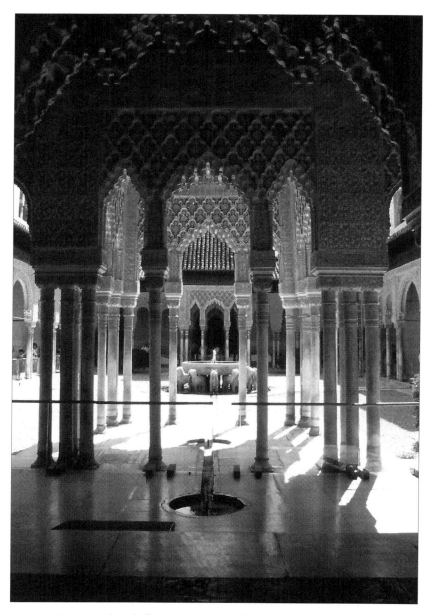

Courtyard with flowing water at Alhambra Palace of Lions.
Photo by the author.

I was immediately enamored by the gentle water flow from the central, circular Fountain of Lions, noting how through tiny, two-inch channels it was directed towards the four corners of the courtyard. To my physician's mind, the narrow channels perfused the courtyard like coronary vessels of the heart.

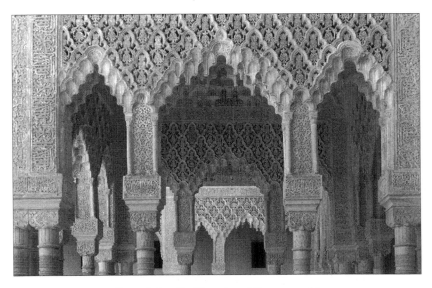

Fractal detail, Alhambra (Shutterstock)

Masculine/feminine balance radiates from the twelve masculine, white marble lions supporting the feminine alabaster circular basin. As the water flows out of the lions' mouths into the courtyard channels, the two energies merge. Scholars generally consider that the four sections of the square courtyard represent the four parts of the world, being fed by the four rivers of paradise. I could sense how, over seven hundred years later, the energy of the space created by these early Islamic artisans is still being amplified and synergized.

Travels to Asia in the mid '90s took my wife and me to Nepal and India. After a month of medical volunteer work in a small village in the Langtang Himalayas of Nepal, we headed south by plane and train to the impressive Taj Mahal, on the banks of the Yamuna River in Agra, India. Departing early one foggy morning from New Delhi, we arrived in Agra in clear blue skies. The ride, along rough train tracks, required a stop en route after a wheel worked loose on one of the passenger cars. We thought we were in for a derailment, but it was averted luckily. Safely in town, we maneuvered around a busy local market and were finally in front of the mausoleum.

My first impression from this monument was divine love. One could see how Mughal emperor Shah Jahan did his best to convey his deep love and sorrow for his wife, who passed while giving birth to his fourteenth child.

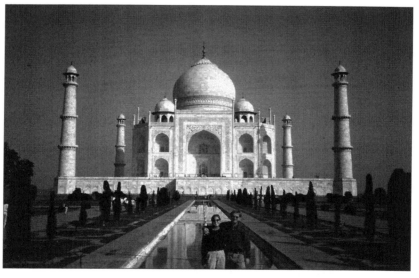

The author and his wife at the Taj Mahal, 1996

Symmetry of the Taj Mahal was visible everywhere, from the teardrop-shaped domes to the four surrounding minaret towers, the four-axis horizontal alignments, and four floors. The reflection pools leading up to the Taj Mahal mirror the symmetry of the massive mausoleum, amplifying its size. Even the moon pools across the Yamuna River capture the dome's reflection, framing it in gardens. Layered like an onion, the dome is capped with a lotus carving. The ornate, artistic detail of inlaid leaves and flowers on the marble faces of the temple further creates an intimate relationship with nature. These features, particularly the lotus pattern throughout the Taj, are its most prominent elements of sacred geometry borrowed from nature.

The masculine/feminine energy unity is also captured through the harmonious integration of the tear-dropped domes into the rectangular base.

In 2016, I traveled to Angkor Wat and the surrounding temples with a meditation group. Our intent was to align with the ancient energies of the temples through meditation and—for planetary healing—to help activate those that were dormant. The size and number of temples far exceeded my expectations. The many temples were commissioned during the reigns of successive rulers, and depending on the beliefs of a king, a given temple may be dedicated to a Hindu deity or Buddha. Even the most ancient temples we visited were constructed with the greatest artisanship, balance, and proportion, equal to that in Angkor Wat, but smaller in scale.

Angkor Wat, the largest temple complex in the world, was built by Khmer King Suryavarman II in Cambodia during the twelfth century AD and dedicated to the Hindu god Vishnu. Suryavarman II and his architects designed it to represent the mystical holy Mount Meru, sacred to Hindu, Jain, and Buddhist cosmology.

This golden mountain in Hindu mythology is the home of deities, and Hindu, Buddhist, and Jain mythology considers it the center of the spiritual, metaphysical, and physical universe.[83] The lotus-bud towers represent the mountain peaks of Mount Meru (see figure). Interestingly, it is oriented to the west, rather than the more traditional eastward alignment of most temples. Perhaps this is to connect it with the mystical mountain. Others feel its design orients it towards Vishnu in India, and of course there are a number of variant theories. Despite this initial dedication to Vishnu, the temple has been more aligned towards Buddhism since the twelfth century. Vishnu is the Hindu god of Protection and Preservation.

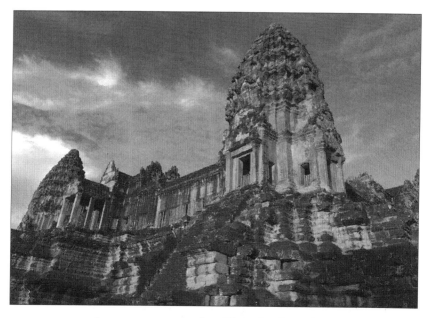

Lotus towers at Angkor. Photo by the author.

Water moats surround the temple complex in a symmetrical manner, with a perimeter wall that runs 2.2 miles and is thought to represent the surrounding ocean.

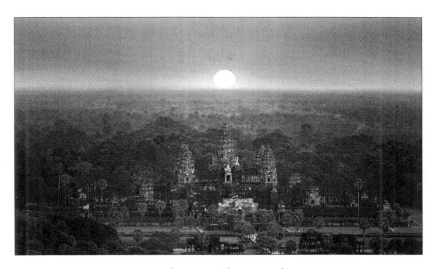

Angkor Wat (Shutterstock)

Combining the encircling ocean with the five lotus peaks of Mount Meru creates one of the most powerful sacred-geometry temples in the world. Many Hindus, Jains, and Buddhists make the sacred pilgrimage around Mount Kailash in Tibet to experience the physical embodiment of the mystical Mount Meru. Jonette Crowley, channel, author, and spiritual adventurer, describes what she experienced leading a pilgrimage around Kailash in 2018: "After doing a three-day pilgrimage around Mount Kailash in Tibet, my 'crystal heart' was activated. This gave me and my entire group the sense that our spiritual hearts were upgraded, connecting us to the crystal Earth star and the cosmos in a unique and powerful way."

Angkor Wat and many other temples mirror Mount Meru, amplifying the energies further. I am thankful to my friend Terry Smith, who made the pilgrimage and placed a Lemurian crystal for me in the sacred Lake Manasarovar, honoring Mount Kailash, which reflects in its waters. The architects of ancient temples and pyramids clearly deployed transformational mathematics, to connect heaven and earth. Lawlor notes three general mathematical processes involved: "the Generative, symbolized by square root of 2, the Formative symbolized by the square root of 3, and the Regenerative symbolized by the square root of 5 and its related function to phi." Architects and astronomers working with these principles helped to geometrically construct and align the temples to the cardinal directions, the stars, and the solstices for optimal spiritual alignment with the gods and beyond. In *Heaven's Mirror* (1998), Graham Hancock—quoting the research of John Grisby, his twenty-five-year-old assistant—hypothesized that the temples around and including Angkor Thom and Angkor Wat align perfectly with the northern constellation of Draco in 10,500 BC.[84]

Similarly, to the west of Cambodia, in their 1994 book, *The Orion Mystery: Unlocking the Secrets of the Pyramids*, Adrian Gilbert and Robert Bauval noted the alignment of the Orion constellation with the great pyramids of Egypt. For what purpose? To activate a resonate field, perhaps even a portal? Was the intent to give a higher resonant field and coherence to the temples and the people living around them? Frequently asserted by sages, ancient and modern, the statements "As above, so below" (and "as the stars align") perhaps were behind these temple/stars alignments.

Similarly, we sometimes hear of the "god within us" being one with the God of the universe. The expression of our DNA has coevolved, or epigenetically shifted, over thousands of years in adapting to the Earth, our solar system, and the broader universe. Our physical and energetic body, all the way down to the subatomic level, mirrors these fractal geometries surrounding us. Tapping deeply into a sacred site's geometry, its alignment to the

stars and energetic positioning on Earth provides a unique opportunity for us to further amplify, and possibly activate our DNA to
the intelligence and interdimensional field of the cosmos.

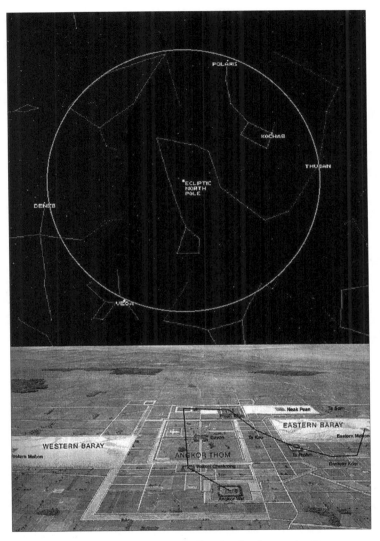

As above, so below. Draco mirrored in Angkor's temple alignments.
Source: "The official Graham Hancock Forum and Astronomy at Angkor" by
Jim Alison—after the copyrighted image in *Heaven's Mirror,* page 127.

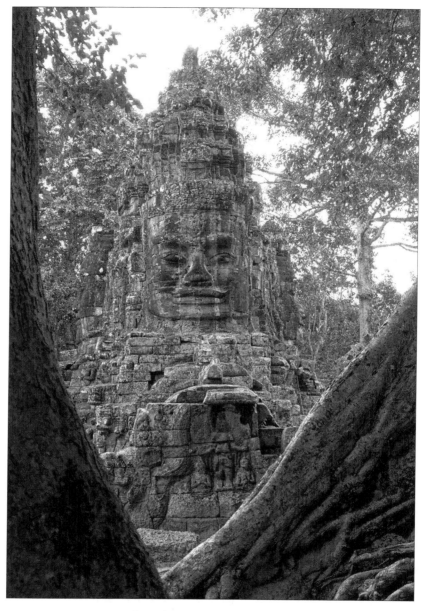

Angkor Thom. Photo by the author.

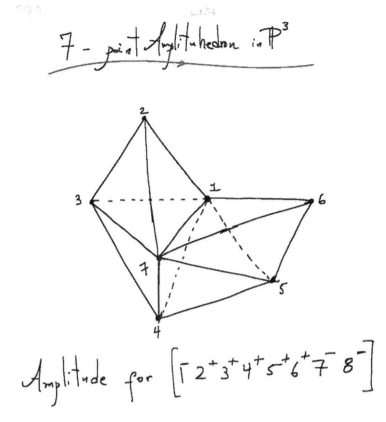

7 – point Amplituhedron in $\mathbb{P}^3$

Amplitude for $\left[\overline{1}\ 2^+ 3^+ 4^+ 5^{-+} 6^+ \overline{7}\ 8^-\right]$

Amplituhedron (a sketch by Nima Arkani-Hamed)

Expanding the concepts of space geometry, particle interactions, and space-time, Nima Arkani-Hamed (a theoretical physicist at the Institute for Advanced Study in Princeton, New Jersey) and his student Jaroslav Trnka (now assistant professor in the Department of Physics, the University of California Davis) introduced in 2013 the *amplituhedron*, a jewel-like geometric structure that enables dramatically simplified calculation of outcomes of particle interactions in some quantum field theories. (See illustration below.) In explaining the significance, senior writer Natalie Wolchover wrote in *Quanta Magazine*: "Beyond making calculations easier or possibly leading the way to quantum gravity, the discovery of the amplituhedron could cause an even more profound shift, Arkani-Hamed said. That is, giving up space and time as fundamental constituents of nature and figuring out how the Big Bang and cosmological evolution of the universe arose out of pure geometry."[85] Extremely importantly, "the revelation that particle interactions, the most basic events in nature, may be consequences of geometry significantly advances a decades-long effort to reformulate quantum field theory, the body of laws describing elementary particles and their interactions."

Further research on the amplituhedron and other complex geometries by astrophysicists will help us better understand our intimate relationship to the universe. I am hopeful to see further astrophysics research analyzing the relationship of geometry and energy flow in the universe compared to our quantum human energy body. Once we discover these deeper relationships, physicians can appreciate and specifically address an imbalanced energy body, rather than simply deploying drugs and surgery.

We are still in the early stages of determining the shape of the universe. Many theories exist, ranging from flat, spherical (positive curvature) to saddle-like shape (negative curvature). As will be discussed and illustrated in the next chapter, in 1984, Russian scientists—Alexi Starobinski and Yakov B. Zeldovich—proposed a three-torus, or doughnut, model as the shape of the universe. A toroid, which has a vortex at both ends, is often visualized as a doughnut, but it's found in many forms, from a smoke ring to an apple to an orange, to plants, to hurricanes, and so on. Determining the shape, geometry, and energy of the universe is important to understanding the subatomic, genotypic (DNA level), and phenotypic (physical body) blueprint of humans. I feel we will be able to transcend most diseases and imbalances once we gain this knowledge.

Arthur M. Young, the designer of Bell Helicopter's first helicopter and author of *The Reflexive Universe*, states, "*The self in a toroidal Universe can be both separate and connected with everything else.*" So, perhaps our human toroidal flow mirrors the energetic flow of the universe too.

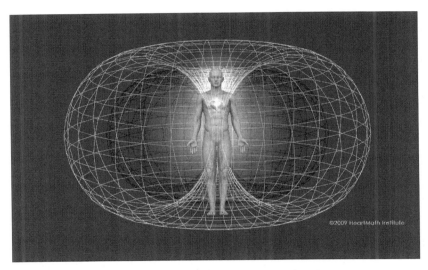

**Human Toroid Field "Electroman" image, used with permission,
© HeartMath Institute**

Unifying these theories, Aikido founder Morihei Ueshiba, in his *New York Times* bestseller *The Art of Peace*, states: "*All things, material and spiritual, originate from one source and are related as if they were one family. The past, present, and future are all contained in the life force. The universe emerged and developed from one source, and we evolved through the optimal process of unification and harmonization.*"[86]

Further travels have brought me to many other unique architectural sites, which would take another book to describe! From the Greek and Roman temples of the Mediterranean, to the Egyptian pyramids, temples along the Nile, Maya and Aztec pyramids of Mexico and Guatemala, Tibetan stupas, Hindu temples of Southeast Asia, to the mystical Inca and pre-Inca sites of Peru and Bolivia—all have sacred geometry, astronomical alignments, and an energy field that is palpable while walking meditatively in and amongst them. This precise geometric construction aligned to the stars, sun, and moon is a common thread amongst these ancient sacred sites. How the megalithic structures such as Sacsayhuaman in Peru were built and aligned without computers, lasers, advanced stone-cutting tools, and cranes is still debated by engineers and archeologists. Modern cranes can only lift 40,000 pounds, a stone 1/10th the size of an estimated 440,000-pound stone at Sacsayhuaman. Obviously, this make it difficult to buy into the archeological theories of ropes and ramps.

Regardless of this mystery and others, simply walking, breathing, and meditating amongst these enigmatic ancient temples and pyramids has undoubtedly epigenetically shifted me to feeling more balanced and connected to the universe.

In summary, by aligning to the geometry of the universe through art and architecture, we are resonating ourselves and our DNA into a healthier state congruent with the order of the cosmos. I believe the ancients were well aware of this, as we seem to have forgotten. We too can facilitate a more multidimensional appreciation of ourselves, our world, and the cosmos when we visit these sites in a mindful state, and not simply seeking a selfie for a social media post. I encourage everyone to explore and experience these gifts awaiting you nearby and around the world.

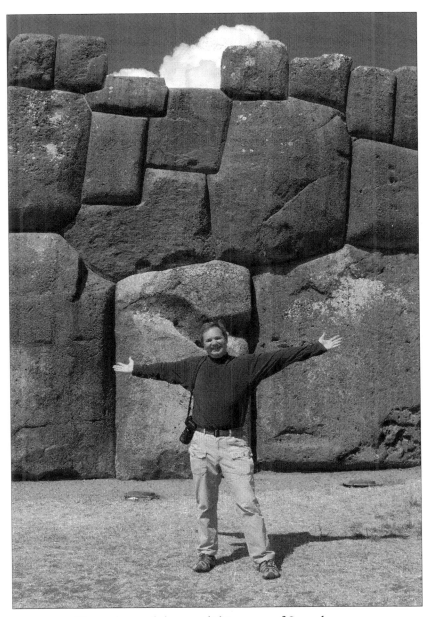

The author and the megalithic stones of Sacsayhuaman
Inca Citadel site, in Cusco, Peru. Stones up to an estimated
200 metric tons (440,000 lbs.) make up the fortress walls,
which need no mortar due to their perfect laser-like articulations.
A modern crane can only lift 40,000 lbs.

Chapter 4

Resonating with the Sacred Geometry of Nature

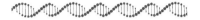

In the '80s I journeyed to Costa Rica for an immersion in tropical plant life and volcanoes with my botany professor and fifteen other students. The patterns of leaves, flowers, and the overlapping branches of the rainforest canopy mesmerized me. In the rainforest, one often drops into a deep primal connection, especially when walking amongst the old-growth trees with their large, supportive buttresses and roots sprawling across the jungle floor. Imaging the mycelial fungal network in the damp forest floor connecting like neurons in our brains deepens one's primal relationship to it even more. I feel this in most forests, but the energy in a rainforest is particularly complex, more ancient and vibrant, teeming with a hundred times more species per acre than anywhere in my Colorado forests. Just 2.47 acres of rainforest "may contain over 750 types of trees and 1,500 species of higher plants."[87]

One afternoon our group was exploring Monteverde's cloud forest, a unique ecosystem in the mountains at 4,600 feet along the continental divide. The preserve receives eight feet of rain annually and is home to the rare, mystical, vibrantly colored bird called quetzal and 400 other bird species, 100 species of mammals, tens of thousands of insect species, and over 2,500 varieties of plants, 420 of which alone are orchids.[88]

As we hiked along the misty, muddy trail, George, our professor, would stop periodically and quench his thirst by squeezing hanging moss into his mouth. I was waiting for a bug to drop in, for entertainment, but no luck! On the upper trail we came upon a tree fern. He explained how tree ferns are some of the most ancient of all plants; they were present during the time of the dinosaurs and are still found in the few surviving rainforests around the world. (See image of tree frond)

Naturally drawn to the center of the spiraling frond, I zoomed in with my Kodachrome 64 film, snapping different angles. Photography has been an amazing creative therapy for me since I was given an SLR by my father when I was fourteen. Framing nature though a lens, setting the right shutter speed and aperture, and perhaps setting up a tripod can seem disruptive, but it takes me into an intimate, spatially analytical mindset that opens a deeper relationship to nature.

As I zoomed in I lost all awareness of the scientific discussion around me and was captivated by the spiral curl in the center of the frond. This curl represents the Fibonacci sequence, a mathematical progression characterized by the fact that every number after the first two numbers is the sum of the two preceding; thus, 1, 1, 2, 3, 5, 8, 13, 21, 34, and so on.[89]

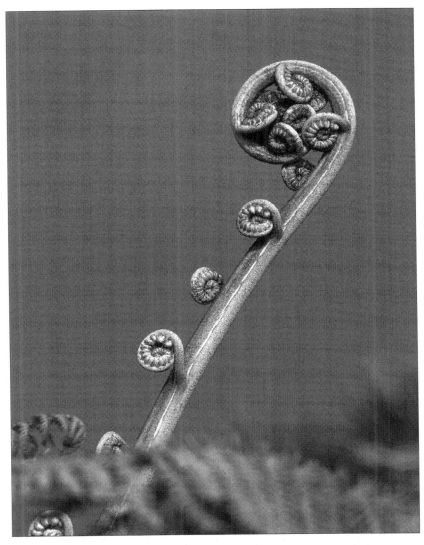

Fibonacci Spirals of fern frond by Sandy Milla on Unsplash

Named after the thirteenth-century Italian mathematician Leonardo Fibonacci, who introduced it to the West in *Liber Abaci* (*The Book of Calculation*, 1202), the Fibonacci sequence approximates the golden spiral and phi ratio, of 1.6180339887. In a never-ending succession, "The ratio of each successive pair of numbers in the sequence approximates Phi (1.618 . . .), as 5 divided by 3 is 1.666 . . . and 8 divided by 5 is 1.60."[90] Known by many names, 1.618 is the "golden number," golden ratio, golden section, or simply "phi."

In Greece, around 300 BC, Euclid, the "father of geometry," was the first to clearly define what we now call "the golden ratio": he stated that

> *A straight line is said to have been cut in extreme and*
> *mean ratio when, as the whole line is to the greater*
> *segment, so is the greater to the lesser.*[91]

Thus, a "golden section" exists when if line AC is cut, line AC is to the greater segment AB as AB is to the smaller segment. In the illustration below, AC is not named. But it is the sections a + b. Dividing the whole top line (AC), into a larger *a* section and smaller *b* section, you get the formula.

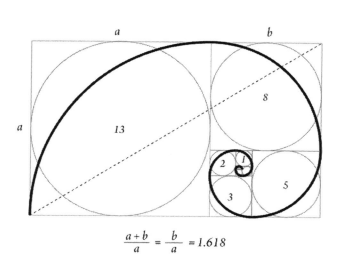

$$\frac{a+b}{a} = \frac{b}{a} = 1.618$$

Golden ratio and Fibonacci sequence (Shutterstock)

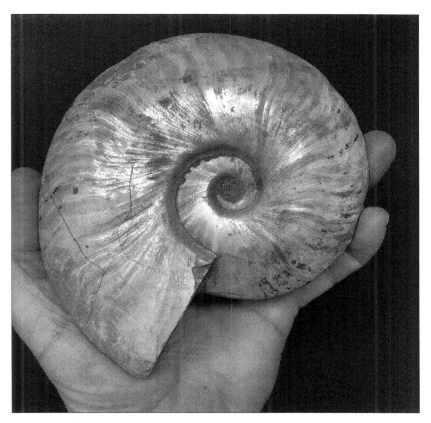

Ammonite fossil with golden ratio/Fibonacci sequence. Photo by the author.

The Renaissance, begun in Italy in the fourteenth century but anticipated at least in the reign of Frederick the Second in the thirteenth century, saw a rediscovery of Greek and Roman antiquity, with pronounced shifts away from medieval taste and institutions, building on preexisting trends. Departing from Byzantine stylization—a Christ of halos and gold leaf, for instance—toward Greek classical naturalism led many artists to study anatomy. Some studied the human form by dissecting unclaimed dead bodies, which were likely to be male. A rare chance to see an exhibit of Leonardo's anatomical drawings opened in Buckingham Palace on May 4, 2012.[92]

Lifelike observation also involved relationship. In the fifteenth-century the Franciscan friar Luca Pacioli, sometimes referred to today as the "Father of Accounting and Bookkeeping," published *The Collected Knowledge of Arithmetic, Geometry, Proportion, and Proportionality*—produced early on, on the Gutenberg press.[93] His second book, *De divina proportione* (*On the Divine Proportion*), came out in 1509 in Venice and propelled our topic forward:

> The subject was mathematical and artistic proportion, especially the mathematics of the golden ratio and its application in architecture. Leonardo da Vinci drew the illustrations of the regular solids in *De divina proportione* while he lived with and took mathematics lessons from Pacioli. Leonardo's drawings are probably the first illustrations of skeletonic solids, which allowed an easy distinction between front and back. The work also discusses the use of perspective by painters such as Piero della Francesca, Melozzo da Forlì, and Marco Palmezzano. As a side note, the "M" logo used by the Metropolitan Museum of Art in New York City is taken from *De divina proportione*.[94]

The Fibonacci sequence is widespread, even sometimes appearing to be ubiquitous. It's found in a pine cone, flowering artichokes, branching limbs of a tree, a nautilus shell, for example, and even in the interval length of your fingertips: "Each section of your index finger, from the tip to the base of the wrist, is larger than the preceding one by about the Fibonacci ratio of 1.618, also fitting the Fibonacci numbers 2, 3, 5 and 8. By this scale, your fingernail is 1 unit in length. Curiously enough, you also have 2 hands, each with 5 digits, and your 8 fingers are each comprised of 3 sections. All Fibonacci numbers!"[95] Look at your arm. The distance from your elbow to wrist is (ideally) roughly 1.618 times that from the wrist to the middle fingertip.[96]

Going deeper within yourself, you find the spiral pronounced in the double helix of your DNA. A cycle (twist) of the DNA double helix measures 21 angstroms wide by 34 angstroms long.[97] A few paragraphs above, we listed 21 and 34 consecutively in the Fibonacci series. Divide them to get their ratio; amazingly, it's 1.6190476, which closely approximates 1.6180339 . . .

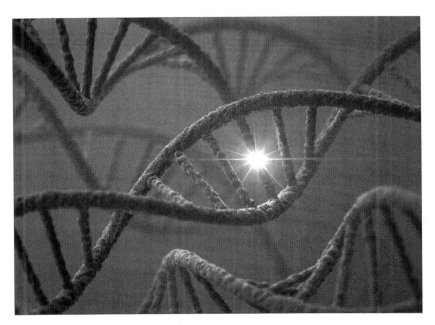

DNA helix (iStock)

New York Times bestseller and international speaker Caroline Myss sees this in the Hindu chakra system as well, in that, she observes, the chakras line up along "a central subtle energy channel . . . the sushumna, which is connected to two crisscrossing channels called the ida and pingala in a pattern that is strikingly similar to the double helix of DNA."[98]

The pineal gland, located near the center of our head, has a pine cone-like anatomy. This small gland is a deep-brain structure, connected with Third Eye perception through its very powerful neural sensitivity, including cells that have photoreceptors similar to those in our retina. The tip is oriented to the heavens, and the structure spirals downward like a pine cone (see image of the gland and its location in the cranium). An illustration in *The Golden Ratio & Fibonacci Sequence* depicts a pine cone, in which the "counter-rotating spirals . . . are in the Fibonacci ratio, in this case 8:13."[99]

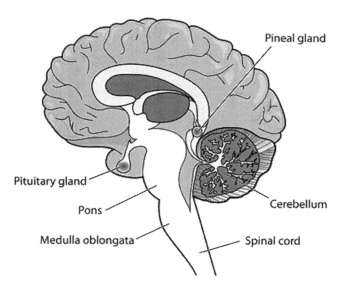

Pineal Gland location in human brain. (Shutterstock)

The courtyard of the Vatican museum has on display the largest known pine cone, the (almost four-meters high) bronze Pigna, from first or second century Rome, which many, including myself, feel is there in recognition of the role of its structure in spiritual connection and intuition. Symbolically, it's compared to the pine-cone shape at Angor Wat or in the staff or Osiris, 1224 BC.[100]

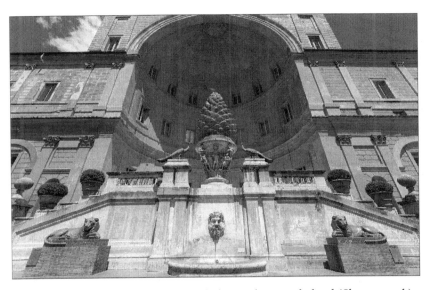

Pigna, Vatican Museum, likely symbolizing the pineal gland (Shutterstock)

As we fly above the rainforest and soar beyond our solar system, we find that we are a small part of another spiral that makes up our Milky Way galaxy. Because we can only photograph the Milky Way from inside our galaxy, NASA explains, "we don't have an image of the Milky Way as a whole. Why do we think it is a barred spiral galaxy, then? There are several clues."[101] I will not stop here to give the clues. But here are a few relevant facts. Our sun is just one in 100 billion or perhaps 400 billion stars in the Milky Way. Over 70 percent of the nearest identified galaxies are spiral. So spirals are within us and around us.

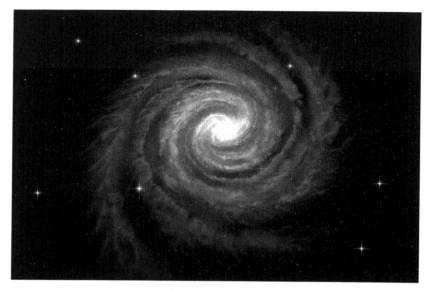

Spiral galaxy (Shutterstock)

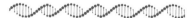

Seeking to understand the relationship of nature and geometry, I contacted internationally recognized sacred geometry artist Francene Hart. She resides on the beautiful Big Island of Hawaii, not far from Kīlauea Volcano, communing and painting in this tropical paradise while keeping an eye on volcanic eruptions. Several years prior I purchased a print of hers titled *Dolphin Merkaba*, which caught my eye in a small gallery in Hawi, an artsy town on the northern end of the island. On a meditative trip to Sedona, I ran across her works in another shop, prompting me to reach out and meet up with her on a recent visit to the Big Island.

In 2017 Simon & Schuster published her diverse palette of mantra-like images in *Sacred Geometry of Nature: Journey on the Path of the Divine*. The publisher introduces her artistic style well, saying:

> Francene reveals how she learned to center her artistic explorations on the intelligence of the heart rather than the intellect, utilizing the wisdom and imagery of Sacred Geometry, reverence for the natural environment, and the interconnectedness between all things as her inspirations. She describes the shamanic lessons that accompanied her discoveries and shaped her understanding of sacred relationships with the self, others, and Mother Earth. She explores how to tap into the energies provided by spirit guides and power animals, like Jaguar, Raven, Octopus, and Dolphin, and explains her profound affinity for the ocean, including her discovery of water consciousness in Hawaii. Offering chronicles of her inspiring travels and transformational encounters around the world, Hart shares her experiences at sacred sites in the Amazon, Central America, Egypt, England, Scotland, Paris, Cambodia, and the Himalayas and how these places influenced her art.

Unless otherwise stated, the paintings in the interview below are by Francene Hart. Over breakfast at Daylight Mind Coffee in Kona she expressed her thoughts on several questions I had for her.

FRED: In your new book, you speak of having a vivid imagination as a child. You say, "There is magic in nature." You also say there is a "hidden order of things." What do you mean? Could you give us an example?

FRANCENE: Most modern cultures have lost connection with the great mysteries. Both the wisdom of the ancients and the intuitive creativity of children have much to reteach us about looking beyond the obvious to what may seem hidden yet holds deeper relevance in our lives.

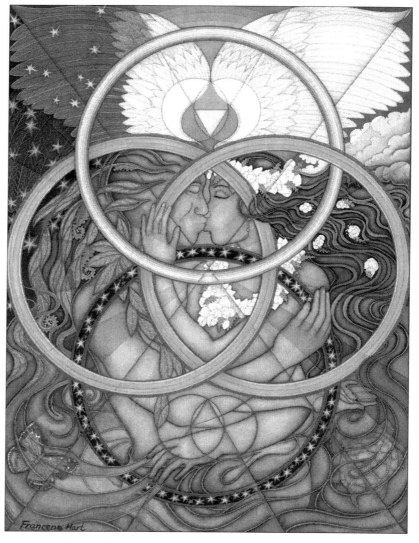

The Kiss by Francine Hart (note the central vesica piscis)

FRED: You also discuss how painting symbols and geometries in mandalas helped catalyze your artistic style. Did you find that natural patterns such as the hexagonal honeycomb, spirals in shells, and the overlapping circles of the *vesica piscis* help you connect and manifest the sacred geometric elements in nature? I like your definition of the vesica piscis, which is "two overlapping spheres with the same radius, intersecting in such a way that the center of each sphere lies on the perimeter of the other."[102]

FRANCENE: Early experiences with mandalas led me to explore symbology that occurs in cultures around the planet throughout history. These were my first steps towards recognizing sacred geometry.

FRED: What are the most effective ways you've found for others to connect to the sacred geometry of nature? Should they sketch plants or animals, or simply meditate in nature?

FRANCENE: How we connect will depend on our natural tendencies. As an artist, I discovered the information encoded in this language of light, and it opened an exciting adventure for me.

The best way I feel for beginners to connect is open eyes and imagination to everything. When observing the patterns in nature, from microscopic to the vastness of the cosmos, you will notice they contain observable geometric patterns. Circles, spirals, triangles, and hexagons are just the start. It is termed a language because it informs us in ways both subtle and profound. Draw, dance, play, ENJOY!

FRED: Excellent tips. What do you mean when you say you discovered information encoded in the language of light? Is that a deeper spiritual or energetic connection with nature that you are tapping into?

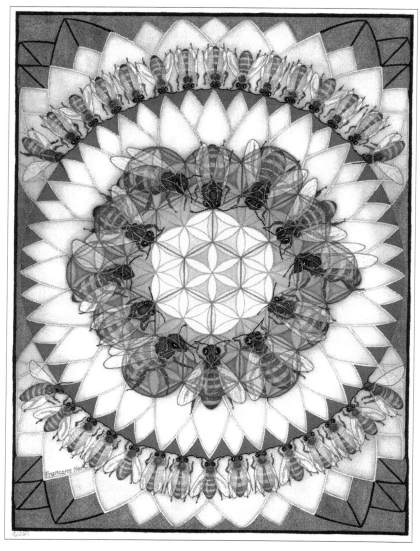

Bee Mandala by Francine Hart (note the central
hexagon and Flower of Life pattern)

FRANCENE: Once the exploration begins, it is truly like looking
into the eyes of creation. Playing in this field helps expand appreciation for our connection with everything.

FRED: Which geometric forms do you feel resonate most deeply with our DNA? Your image titled *Rainbow DNA* has always intrigued me.

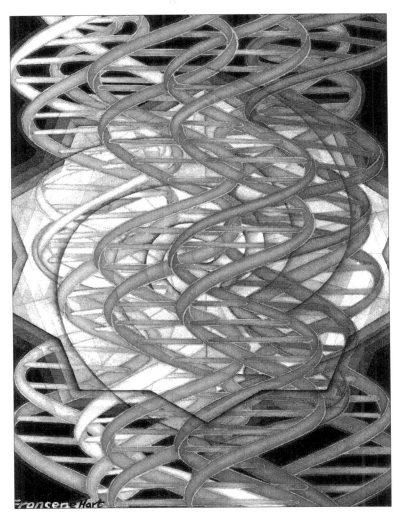

Rainbow DNA by Francine Hart

FRANCENE: Our DNA utilizes the golden spiral, with its phi ratio, to form the wave that spins our genetic code. The ratio also exists in many of the configurations associated with sacred geometry.

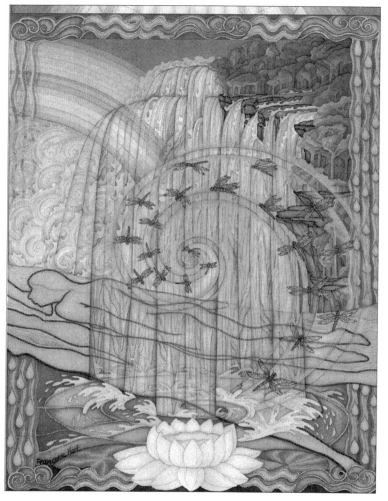

Fresh Splash by Francene Hart (illustrates the
golden spiral and Fibonacci sequence)

FRED: Can sacred geometry enhance, balance, and open chakras?
For example, when looking at paintings, nature, or the architectural elements of temples, cathedrals, and other sacred places?

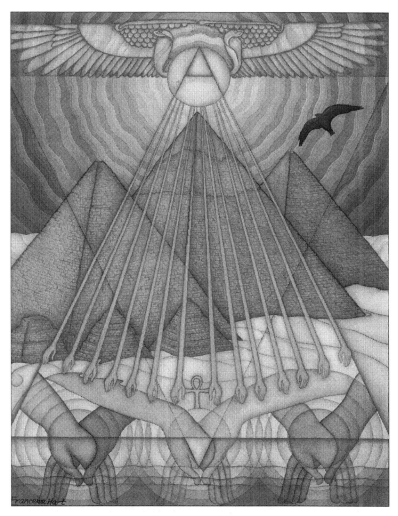

Pharonic Fusion by **Francine Hart**

FRANCENE: Perfections within these configurations is seeded deep within our DNA. Developing an understanding of the wisdom field held within these beautiful patterns can become an instinctive path towards both self-awareness and the understanding that we are all one. Whether approached as a means to create balance or an opening to our divine nature, which our chakras exemplify, there is assistance available within the information. Chakras are spinning wheels of light containing energy and information that helps us understand who we are.

I have traveled extensively to sacred sites and temples. I have deeply felt the intelligence contained in these places and been moved to my core by the beauty held therein.

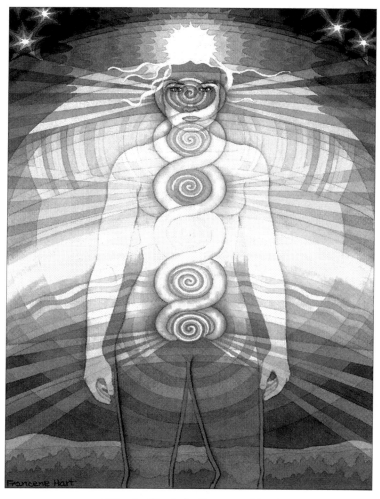

Wheels of Light by **Francene Hart**

FRED: When you refer to understanding the "wisdom field," is that a competency people may develop as they recognize the higher orders of these plant patterns and geometries?

FRANCENE: Yes. Each of us has an intuitive ability to recognize higher orders. Allowing ourselves to tune into these geometries and vibrations is a gift we can give our hearts.

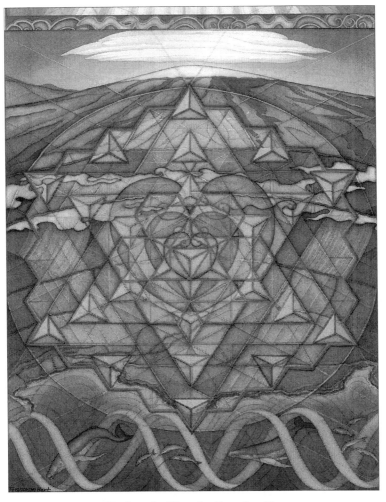

Healing the Heart by Francine Hart

FRED: I see that you grasp the shamanic forces and intelligence of "power animals." I've had the insight that dolphins and whales, for instance, may communicate to each other in 3-D or a holographic way. Do you also feel that's the case?

FRANCENE: Absolutely! I have experienced this both visually and energetically with the dolphins and whales. We have much to learn from our cetacean friends. Here's an example.

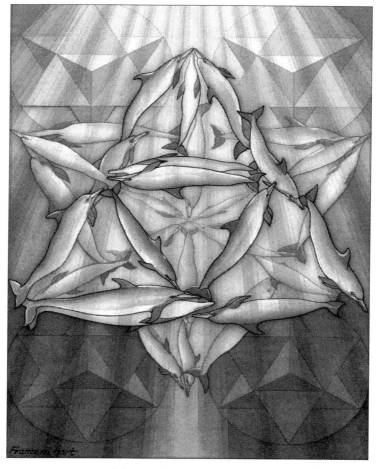

Dolphin Merkaba by Francene Hart

Swimmers often tell stories of shifting dimensions or even moving through time as they swim with dolphins. One day we witnessed them forming the star tetrahedral configuration associated with the Merkaba. In sacred geometry this form is known to be a vehicle of multidimensional travel. Connecting in this fashion confirms a form of interspecies communication.

FRED: I have read that you experimented in your younger years with psychedelic plants as a consciousness-altering technique. Can such plant medicines as ayahuasca, San Pedro, and psilocybin help us connect to the sacred geometry of nature and the universe?

FRANCENE: Plant medicine was certainly helpful to me as a gateway for experiencing other dimensions and initiated a life-defining experience in which I knew myself as part of every molecule in the universe. It was profound, yet once that door was opened, I felt no personal need to replicate the experience.

I now find that meditation, visualization, and yoga are more in alignment with my path.

FRED: Do you believe that sacred sites like Cambodia's Angkor Wat or powerful geologic sites—for example, Ayers Rock, or Sedona's Boynton Canyon—can create a geometric resonate field, such as a vortex, that can positively impact our energy field and chakras?

FRANCENE: Yes, where we live, work and travel, as well as our chakras, are intimately affected by geometric resonance. People with subtle energy sensitivity will feel the shifts immediately. Finding a place on the planet that resonates with who you are, is helpful in feeling and being in balance with earth energies.

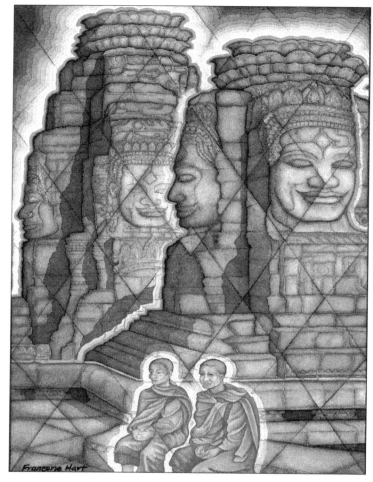

Byon Faces by Francine Hart (Angkor Wat complex)

FRED: Do you feel the ancients used sacred geometry to heal and connect to the other dimensions?

FRANCENE: Many of the ancients knew far more than we do today. I believe we are only beginning to understand the vastness that came before us, and the layers of wisdom that are continually being revealed. Sacred geometry is a wonderful tool to help us grow out of our limited, historical view of reality.

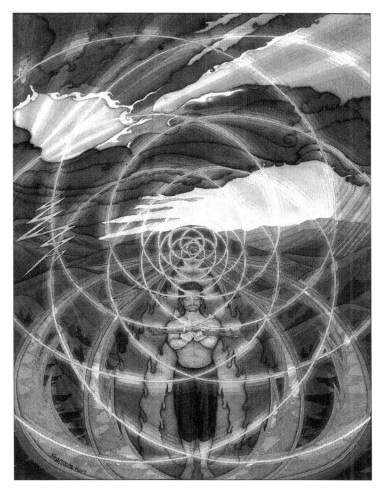

Piercing the Veil by Francene Hart

FRED: I agree. Like you, I've seen the integration of nature into the sacred geometry of their ancient temples via reliefs or paintings of plants and animals. This is visible all over the world, especially in in Egypt, Turkey, Greece, Cambodia, Nepal, Peru, and Guatemala. My favorite being the more recent excavation of Gobekli Tepe ("potbelly hill"), which predates the Egyptian pyramids and has stone carvings of birds and reptiles visible on a Stonehenge-like circle. All of this creates a palpable flow of energy. In fact, I've experienced what I'll call "activations" at many sites. Initially, I thought I was crazy when I sensed these, but after discussing with other spiritual adventurers, I've discovered this phenomenon is common to those who meditate, and don't just photograph at a site. My most memorable was at Palenque (a Maya city) several years back. I had traveled alone to this remote location in Chiapas (Mexico) to experience this mystical site nestled in a misty rainforest with waterfalls, and the echo of howler monkeys in the hillsides. As I meditated at a small pyramid, I felt an intense rush of energy flowing from my sacrum up my spine, bringing in visuals of the community when it was inhabited. The "activation" thus included not only a kundalini-like flow of energy but as well an informational download. Sometimes there is a tingling between my brow that then flows down my spine. This, in my opinion, may represent energetic flow through the Third Eye and pineal gland, which can then flow to the other chakras.

Doubtless, you could write a book on activations you've received, and how they've stimulated much of your artwork! Thank you for all that you've done to help me and others see this relationship through your beautiful nature-inspired, mandala-like paintings. Additional gratitude, not only for contributing to the field of art, but also for helping others resonate with the code and geometry of nature, thus energetically and spiritually connecting us deeper with Gaia and the universe surrounding us.

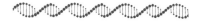

To dive deeper into our relationship with sacred geometry and how it may activate our DNA, I interviewed Gregory Hoag, an expert sacred geometer, who founded Metaforms, which makes 3-D geometric forms and jewelry.

Fortunately, Greg lives up the road from me in the foothills of the Colorado Rockies. On a spring day in 2017, I made the hour drive up to his beautiful mountain home north of Boulder. He and his wife, Gail, have created an energy field—including vortexes—that when walking around their property anyone can quite palpably feel. Helping produce the field are his six-foot-tall sacred-geometric copper sculptures, with many more inside. Over a three-hour videotaped interview, Greg roamed through his vast knowledge. I've narrowed down the interview to the pearls of our discussion. For reference, I've also included the images of geometric shapes discussed.

FRED: Which geometric forms resonate with and potentially activate our DNA?

GREGORY: Everything organic, growing, and alive is working with the phi ratio, or golden mean proportion, which is a relationship equal to 1.618 . . . , which results when the long length of the geometric shape is divided by the short length. The three periods after the number denote that the number sequence never ends. In mathematics, 1.618 . . . is considered an irrational number, but as a geometry it exists quite nicely in our reality. The DNA double helix is often modeled by stacking dodecahedrons, which have 12 pentagonal sides. The pentagon is the one polygon where every internal angle is reflected in triangles of phi ratio relationships.

Axial View of
DNA Double Helix

Dodecahedral Rotation
of DNA Double Helix

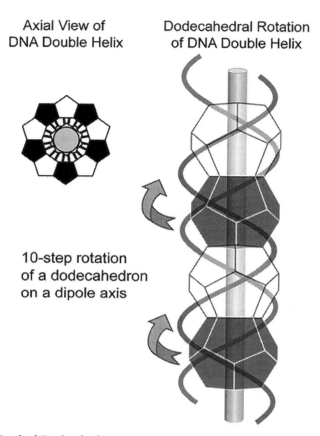

10-step rotation
of a dodecahedron
on a dipole axis

Stacked Dodecahedrons rotating around central axis, model-
ing the DNA double helix. Credit: Mark White, MD.

Thus, the Star Dodecahedron, where the height of the five-sided pyramid on each face of the dodecahedron is 1.618 . . . times the base length, is a great example of a DNA-activating geometry.

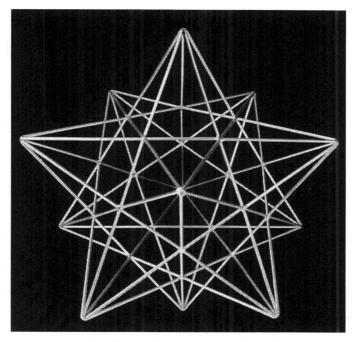

Star Dodecahedron by Greg Hoag

It resonates with the higher Christ body of consciousness (compassion and love) and works with *opening the heart chakra,* the doorway to higher self. These important added elements are needed to properly stimulate DNA in alignment with Divine purpose.

Over twenty-five years ago Dr. Glen Rein tested some of our geometries and found they had a direct effect on DNA. Today he is conducting experiments with the Merkabah of Oneness,

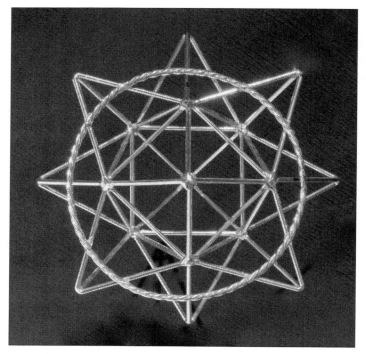

Merkabah of Oneness by Greg Hoag

which is proving to have the strongest effect on unwrapping and "re-zipping" DNA. In form it is similar to a Metatron's Cube turned inside out, which creates a higher-order influx of energy into the physical dimension. But it is always important to couple human intent with the movement of the geometries.

Spinning these forms—at a very precise speed with an added frequency in the megahertz range on a new motor that we have developed—creates a pulsing coherent field that interacts with DNA because of geometric resonance. I think we can leave this image of motor one out.

This is in the same way that a "C" tuning fork will begin to vibrate when a "C" tone is played. Physical geometry becomes the coalescing resonant antenna for the higher-vibrational realms of sound, light, gravity, magnetism, and the higher analogs of the entire electromagnetic spectrum.

FRED: So we see only a tiny fraction of the universe and yet in terms of resonance we tap into much more of it. Walking over your property, passing these sculptures, we sense something of our place in the universe. "Mystics through time have equated [the platonic solids] to various states of consciousness."[103] When you use the phrase "DNA-activating geometry," what do you mean? How does physical geometry activate DNA?

GREGORY: In the case of DNA, this field catalyzes the organized flow of photons, which are responsible for the creation and function of DNA molecules. It has been proven in numerous scientific studies that DNA communicates through photon transfer, what one might call the language of light.

FRED: What is your interpretation of the term "junk DNA"?

GREGORY: Modern science has been stunned by the fact that of the billions of chemical reactions needed to run our bodies, only 1.5 percent of our DNA is used to create them. Thus, the remaining 98.5 percent was labeled "junk DNA," because its function was not understood or recognized. If one were to lay all of this "junk DNA" end to end, it would stretch almost 14 billion miles. The universe doesn't waste energy. It is conservative, precise, and extremely practical in all of its creations. In the case of this disproportionately large amount of DNA, its purpose is in part to be an antenna system linking us to our multidimensional selves through the language of Light. This is also why the process of working with geometries, frequencies, light, and intent is so effective at interacting with our bodies' primary interdimensional communication system—DNA.

FRED: Interesting, yes, and much has changed on this issue of "junk DNA" since the 1970s. In the last few years, scientists have begun to find uses for it. For instance, in 2012 they were discovered to be genetic "switches, signals, and signposts embedded like runes throughout"—as reported in *Scientific American*—"the entire length of the human DNA." In that interview, Ewan Birney, of the European Bioinformatics Institute, who researched "junk DNA," said the term should be retired, "totally expunged from the lexicon. . . . I am now convinced that it's just not a very useful way of describing what's going on." Birney also explained that more of the DNA is used for regulating genes than for protein coding, which was the original purpose assigned to it. He said the amount of DNA used for regulating genes could be as high as 20 percent![104] In 2018 the news is exciting indeed. A Princeton article called "Imaging in Living Cells Reveals How Junk DNA Turns On a Gene" describes how video captured evidence "showing how pieces of DNA once thought to be useless can act as on-off switches for genes."[105]

I feel confident that many more on-off switches, once termed "junk DNA," will be identified. Discovering how we might turn them on or off through mindfulness and stimulate them via sacred geometric forms will make for a fascinating future in epigenetics. Perhaps holding these Metaforms and flowing deeper into the geometry, just as we observe abstract art, will help communicate to us the building blocks of the unseen interdimensional universe, as described in the entanglement theory. Who knows what new theories of the universe could be generated by this too!

The entanglement theory, dubbed by Einstein as "spooky action at a distance," is a quantum effect where one particle gets connected to another such that an action on one will affect the other. This can happen even at large distances. Typically cited as involving subatomic particles, *it was recently documented in two, 3-millimeter-wide diamond crystals,* spaced fifteen centimeters apart, at room temperature. University of Oxford professor Ian Walmsley, who led the international research team that published their study in *Science* in 2011, noted that "In fact, the universe doesn't know which diamond is vibrating!"[106] As another team member, physicist Joshua Nunn of Oxford University, further explained, "The diamonds are entangled, with one vibration shared between them, even though they are separated in space. We could use a similar technique to measure the diamonds and determine that this was the case."[107]

Speaking of entangled, I can often feel a field of subtle energy as I walk by the large geometric forms around your house. Just as tiny diamonds are geometric crystalline forms, one has to wonder if, beyond our 3-D perceptions, larger geometric forms such as yours may entangle us in the energies they may be aligning with.

Gregory, how would you contrast curved or spiral forms with the more angular forms found in the platonic solids?

GREGORY: When the angular forms spin, they create curves. And as they move through time and space, spirals are formed. The angular masculine is at the core of the softer feminine outer expression as it moves in real time. With the spinning forms that we use, it is important to note that the flavor and the focus of the energy shifts, depending on the point you spin it from and the direction of spin. The physical, spiraling expression of the DNA double helix is a reflection of the spiraling energetic flow that created it.

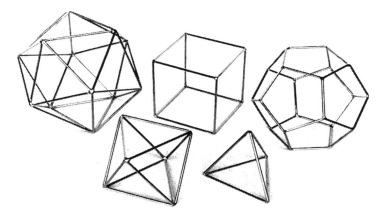

The Platonic Solids by Greg Hoag

FRED: You mean *As Above, So Below?* The multidimensional mirroring of our physical double helix?

GREG: Yes, I consider them our DNA antenna systems. We have learned to activate the potential energy of these DNA antenna systems by spinning three-dimensional geometries, coupled with specific energy components at the proper revolutions per minute.

Furthermore, it is important to note that even though we see a static angular form, as in the platonic solids that you mentioned, acting as antenna systems, these forms attract and move energy on the higher-dimensional levels. This movement is in a toroidal fashion through many different points of the form simultaneously. A torus is shaped like a doughnut, with the outer tube constantly twisting inward or outward depending on which side you are viewing.

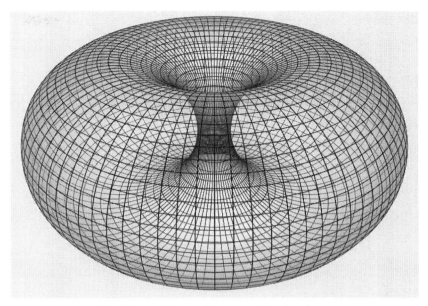

The Torus—Nassim Haramein Facebook page

All of the energy flows it generates are curved and spiraling. If we were capable of witnessing the full dimensional spectrum (by that, I mean the full multidimensionality of our universe), we would see the 3-D geometry acting as the angular "bones" of the higher-dimensional curves and spirals of the feminine, flowing energy. The masculine catalyzes and supplies the impetus, and the feminine informs and directs the flow of photonic energy.

FRED: Thanks for explaining the impact of movement on angular geometric forms. I observed the morphing of a roughly two-foot-tall metallic Merkabah as it went from stationary to spinning powered by a small electric motor, while in a meditation group a few years ago. The angular tetrahedrons quickly shifted to a smooth upper and lower cone as they reached a certain speed. We could feel it emitting a more balanced masculine and feminine energy while it was spinning. Drunvalo Melchizedek and others have powerful YouTube meditations and demonstrations of this form morphing and what you are describing.

GREGORY: Working with subtle energies is unchartered territory for most people, so we suggest that they open to higher guidance as they work with these sacred geometries to help them direct the energies appropriately. Also, the most critical aspect of the process is the understanding that the spinning form creates the field and offers a coherent energy input. It is up to the receivers whether or not they choose—in free will—to step into that field and accept the opportunity for change.

FRED: Can crystals and crystalline structure resonate with our DNA?

GREGORY: Some crystalline structures resonate better than others. Crystals with naturally occurring six-sided displays resonate the best, because their internal molecular structure is made up of spiraling tetrahedrons. These long, spiral vortexes of molecules perfectly duplicate and repeat untold numbers of times. This offers a geometric antenna system on the micro-level magnified many, many times, thus forming long, spiraling geometric pathways for energy to flow in a coherent fashion, amplifying the effects. For this reason, someone sensitive to subtle energies can often feel the vibration of a crystal, and even direct it by conscious interaction.

FRED: Beautiful. Perhaps that's why myself and others feel the energy in places like Sedona and Shasta, which contain high levels of crystalline bedrock, or even working with smaller crystals on the body for energetic healing/balancing. I also enjoy placing crystals to honor and activate sacred places, as pictured below. So why is the number six so important?

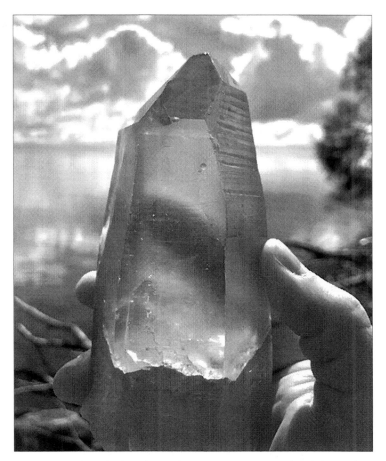

Lemurian crystal placed at Lake Rotorua, New Zealand, by author

GREGORY: In a greater sense, six is the numeric archetype that is the container for our space/time continuum, with the six-pointed star being a symbol for the blending of masculine and feminine, heaven and earth and the heart center, which blends the upper three and lower three chakras.

Some of this springs from the 12/60 base system that human beings have used since the ancient Sumerians. All aspects of our time-keeping are multiples of six: the sacred years used by the Mayans,

Egyptians, and thirty other ancient cultures were 360-day years; with twelve 30-day months in a year; 24 hours in a day (2+4=6); 60 minutes in an hour and 60 seconds in a minute. When properly viewed, the spiraling dodecahedron, which makes up the geometry of the DNA molecule, also has a 6-sided display, as do all of the platonic solids. In fact, all geometries are important multiples of 6—with our basic unit of surface measure, the square, containing 360 degrees, which is 6 x 6 (with the added zero not altering the reduced harmonic). We also see this with the 360 degrees of a circle used for describing all the angles of creation.

FRED: Can you comment on the sacred geometry architecture of the ancients?

GREGORY: Unlike today, almost all ancient cultures knew the importance of reflecting creator in their creations. Sacred geometry as a measure of creating relationship with the natural world was firmly entrenched in each culture's existence—their space/time continuum.

Stonehenge was constructed over 5,000 years ago by moving twenty-five-ton blocks of stone over 150 miles to link with the cycles of time and the movement of the heavens on a sacred site that had been used for eons because of its energetic flow. It is a classic example of ancient architecture demonstrating the squaring of the circle. The pyramids at Giza generated large fields of transformational energies, and in modern times the pyramid shape was the first form to make us aware that shape does affect the environment, with its energy flow. It further reflected the same squaring of the circle seen at Stonehenge. The Greek temples reflected the natural order of creation and were constructed by a civilization that became a blueprint for our present-day growth in science, politics, and philosophy. And the sacred geometry found in Renaissance churches vibrationally raised our spirit into connection with the Divine ethers.

FRED: How does the energy of the Egyptian pyramid compare to other pyramid forms, such as the six-sided ones?

GREGORY: There were many different pyramid angles, but the Great Pyramid at Giza in Egypt is the one most commonly referenced.

My guidance indicates that the Egyptian pyramidal shapes are no longer of the value they once were. There are shapes much more relevant to the spiritual evolution of human beings today, and the focus of my guidance has been toward raising consciousness. The six-sided Aquarian Pyramid 2012 that I have created is one such form that offers higher dimensional connections than the traditional square-based pyramid. The six-sided pyramid is also much more dynamic and integrative in its energy flow, which catalyzes greater transformative potential.

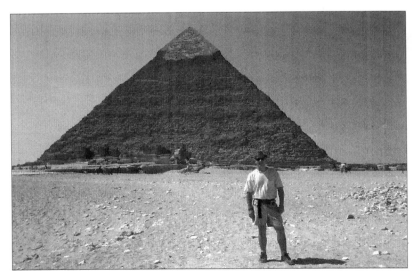

The author at the Great Pyramid, 1996

FRED: Can you comment on the vesica piscis, often found on the façades of medieval and Gothic cathedrals?

GREGORY: The vesica piscis is formed when two circles overlap such that each circle's edge is touching the center of the opposite circle. This convex-lens shape has been referred to as the divine womb that gives birth to everything else. The number 1, a symbol for Unity, is unknowable, infinite in scope, as in the example that all numbers contain 1, but when divided by 1 you only see the original number, not 1. To move into expression in this dimension, Unity divides into 2—duality. The even numbers are feminine; thus, it is through the feminine aspect that the masculine initiating force is first expressed in our reality. This is also why the feminine is gaining in importance today, as we rise in spiritual understanding and are moving back toward Unity through the doorway and understanding of the feminine.

The vesica piscis is within the seed of the Flower of Life geometry and mathematically gives rise to all the different roots and geometries. It is the third element created, formed from Mother Duality and Father Unity. As a 3, it is masculine in nature; Jesus as the son was often portrayed in the center of this form on the façade of Renaissance and medieval cathedrals.

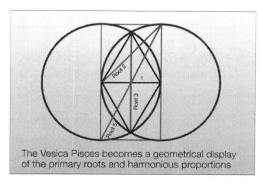

The Vesica Pisces becomes a geometrical display of the primary roots and harmonious proportions

The Vesica Piscis (Pisces) by Greg Hoag

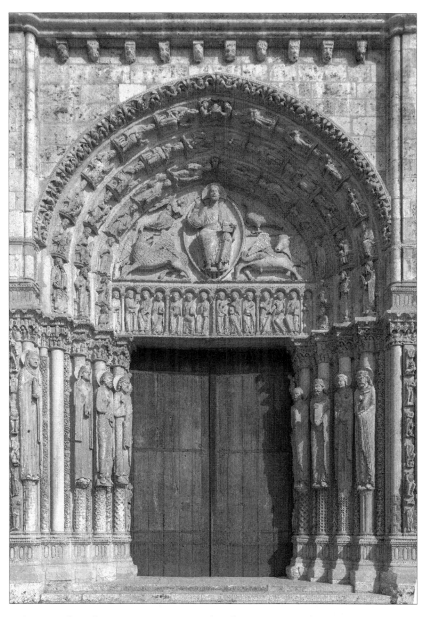

Christ within the Vesica Piscis (completed 1170), central portal of the west
facade (Portail Royal), Chartres Cathedral, France (Shutterstock)

Three, the trinity, is the most powerful, catalytic of all the first nine numbers. Even the six-pointed star, which describes our space/time continuum, is a composite of one triangle over another = 3 + 3.

FRED: Thanks for expanding on the vesica piscis. It's great to have perspective from you and the artist Francine Hart, whom I interviewed earlier. Can you expand on Divine Feminine and Masculine properties inherent in sacred geometry?

GREGORY: As I just shared, the six-pointed star is a composite of two triangles. One points upward towards Father Sky and is masculine in nature. The second, downward-pointing triangle delivers us toward Mother Earth. The sky holds the radiating and catalytic Sun, offering the energetic seed for all creation in the form of the photon/Light. All of these metaphoric elements are properties of the projective masculine force.

Mother Gaia is much more than the receiver of this energy. She forms and directs it toward its greatest expression. She grounds it, grows it to completion, and sustains it until its time for dissolution, which is also her role. She is the gravitational aspect of creation known as Love. In the manifest universe the dance between the masculine and the feminine comes down to the dance between Light and Love.

Human beings have grown very out of balance on this planet, diminishing the important role of the feminine over many thousands of years. The time of separation from the whole is ending. The rise of the Divine Feminine is upon us as a necessary aspect to embrace if we are to survive and evolve to a higher level of consciousness.

FRED: I agree. I think the rise of the Divine Feminine is also creating unrest with those who don't resonate or understand it, particularly with the current leadership in our country. Perhaps as society awakens and comprehends this interrelationship exemplified by sacred geometric principles of balance, we can heal without resorting to polarized anger towards one another. Can you also comment on the importance of the number 108?

GREGORY: First, I would like to respond to your comment about the unrest being created by the rise of the Divine Feminine. We are in a time of transformation, when Love will be able to flow more freely and positively transform, which is the nature of the Mother energy. Where there are unresolved issues, emotional fears that we often refer to as blockages in the body, we will feel discomfort and dis-ease as this mounting flow of Love increases the pressure to bring impediments within each of us to the Light for dissolution and healing.

I assume this question about the number 108 is because we were talking before our taping about all of the different religions that used the same number of prayer beads in their malas.

FRED: Yes, I was seeking more clarity on the 108-count mala. I've always been curious since Perba Sherpa, who helped guide me in the Everest region in 2000, gifted me an old yak bone and a turquoise mala, which I counted and contemplated.

GREGORY: This is a very interesting topic, because 108 prayer beads are on the malas of the Tibetan and Chinese Buddhists, the Taoists, Hindus, and Sikhs. Roman Catholics use a rosary of exactly half that—54 beads. Many ancient Roman temples had 108 columns supporting their roofs, and Islam recognizes that 108 refers to God. Especially in Hinduism, one sees it everywhere: 108 gopis, 108 holy places, 108 Upanishads, and it goes on and on, but no one really has a clear understanding of why. The reasoning is often circular, where we simply see more places it shows up— like 54 letters in the Sanskrit alphabet or 54 intersections in the Sri Yantra. The ancient ruins of Angkor Wat have 5 gates, with the entering avenues bordered by 54 statues on each side—for a total of 108 per road—and 540 stone deities overall.

These same numbers, along with their relationship to the precession of the equinoxes—a 25,920-year cycle—have been spread throughout the world since the great flood, 9,600 years ago. Information from an advanced civilization shared by the survivors of that cataclysm has made its way through time and many cultures as *numbers* of objects. A sound way of keeping encoded information intact and hidden, but obviously it was *not the essence* of the information to be conveyed. Matter (objects) is a very small percentage of reality, as the majority of reality (99.99999 percent as defined by science) is energy. To understand energy, we need to define the *space* (energy) *between* objects, which relates to angles and thus degrees.

FRED: Every year there are so many numerological and geometric correlates being discovered amongst these advanced ancient civilizations. Some scholars—for example, Nassim Haramein—are noting the relationships between sacred geometry and astrophysics. Haramein recently speculated that the I Ching's alignment with 64 may tie into the geometry of space and the universe. This ancient Chinese divination system, he observes, probably predates recorded history in China. Some of his thought, as explained by his Resonance Science Foundation, is below:

From Wikipedia: "The text of the I Ching is a set of oracular statements represented by 64 sets of six lines each called hexagrams (卦 guà). Each hexagram is a figure composed of six stacked horizontal lines (爻 yáo), each line is either Yang (an unbroken, or solid line), or Yin (broken, an open line with a gap in the center). With six such lines stacked from bottom to top there are 26 or 64 possible combinations, and thus 64 hexagrams represented. The solid line represents yang, the creative principle. The open line represents yin, the receptive principle."

Nassim Haramein looked at the hexagrams of the I Ching and analyzed the simple geometry represented by the lines, taking their meaning more as literal geometric information and less as symbolic.

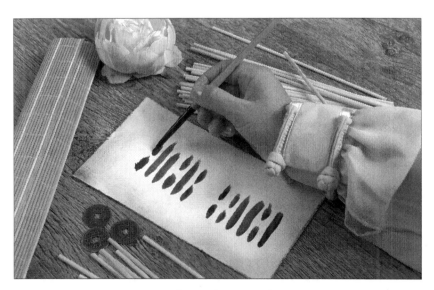

I Ching (Shutterstock)

If you want to build the geometry of the structure of the space that is everywhere in the universe, which is an infinite tetrahedral array, you begin with the first octave of what becomes an infinite fractal division of the space in a perfectly balanced state: a set of 64 tetrahedrons. At 64 tetrahedrons you have what [inventor/visionary] Buckminster Fuller called the "vector equilibrium," also called the cube octahedron (8 tetrahedrons pointing inward) inside a second cube octahedron that is twice as large made of a total of 64 tetrahedrons: an octave.

To get to 64 tetrahedrons, you bring together 8 star tetrahedrons. Each star tetrahedron is made from a tetrahedron pointing up and another polarized pointing downward—creating what is also commonly known as a Merkaba.

Nassim Haramein noticed the only "3D" geometry you can make with 6 solid lines is a tetrahedron, and in order to make the second tetrahedron of a star tetrahedron you would need 6 broken lines to pass through the lines of the first tetrahedron. Nassim decoded the I Ching by showing how 6 solid lines and 6 broken lines are both the building blocks of the I Ching and that of a star tetrahedron.

Thus, the I Ching encodes the most fundamental geometric information you need to build the geometry of the universe! [108]

GREGORY: Before we move on I need to respond to what you stated by Nassim. I respect what he has to share, but again I would like to point out that the universe always conserves energy and moves toward simplicity and the most concise distillation of the fractal seed. An octave means 8, not—8 x 8. As you shared, the Cube Octahedron is made up of 8 tetrahedrons and 64 tetrahedrons, which simply creates a duplication and expansion of the original Cube Octahedron. If you cut the Cube Octahedron in half and flip the outside toward the center, you have a Star Tetrahedron with eight tetrahedronal tips. Where Nassim pointed out that six of the lines forming the Star Tetrahedron were broken as they crossed the first six lines of the original one, this also has the effect of disrupting the energy that creates a flow between the crossed points forming an octahedron in the center. Energy also flows off the tips of each outwardly pointing tetrahedron connecting with the three nearest tips forming a cube. This form has come to be known as Metatron's Cube, and it is the seed fractal of the physical universe. If one stacks 8 Metatron's Cubes to form a large Cube, then you get the form Nassim is referencing, with 64 tetrahedrons. To complete the progression of the seed fractal of Metatron's Cube moving into the dodecahedron and the phi ratio actually involves half of 64, or 32, but this is too large a story for this chapter.

Now, back to the importance of angles. You said, "To understand energy, we need to define the *space* (energy) *between* objects, which relates to angles and thus degrees." Do certain angles and ratios resonate with DNA more effectively?

GREGORY CONTINUED: The first question you asked me in this dialogue was, what forms resonate with DNA? And I said, forms that exhibit the phi ratio of 1.618 . . . The polygon that works with the phi ratio in all the angles it generates is the pentagon. Each of the 5 internal angles on the outside of the form is 108 degrees, and the total of all 5 angles is 540 (when looking at the harmonics of numbers, zeros are disregarded, so here is one source of 54 and 108).

If internally connecting all outside corners with lines, then one creates a pentagram—five-pointed star—which creates two different triangles: a triangle with 108–36–36 degrees and a triangle with 36–72–72 degrees. Both of these triangles are the only triangles that exist where the long side divided by the short side equals 1.618 . . . , phi. We spoke about the importance of the trilogy as the activating force of this dimension, and here we are witnessing two of the most important triangles of biological creation.

Earlier, we also mentioned the 360-degree internal angles of the square and circle. When multiplied by 72, they equal the length of the great year/precession of the equinoxes = 25,920 years created by the wobble of the Earth's axis. The 720 internal degrees of the hexagon times 36 equals the great year, as well as the 1,080 internal degrees of the octahedron times 24, which is 1/3 of 72. Each of these numbers reduces to 9, demonstrating completion on the physical and doorways to the higher divine order. Also, they reduce to 9 in an interesting pattern, using all of the numbers beneath 9. The lower-valued 1 combines with the higher 8 for 108 degrees; then higher 7 combines with lower 2 for 72 degrees; next, following this oscillating pattern, we find 36 and then 54 degrees. Did you also notice that all of the internal sums and multipliers of many other polygons work with the numbers of the angles found only within the pentagon and its phi ratio triangles?

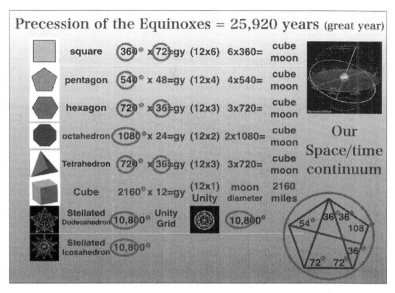

Polygon/pentagon angles in relationship
to space-time and 108 by Greg Hoag

Even the moon is resonant, with a diameter of 2,160 miles that equals the number of degrees in our basic unit of measure: the cube.

FRED: Let's see: a cube has twenty-four 90-degree angles; 24 x 90 = 2,160.

GREGORY: It becomes more intriguing when you realize that the moon's radius is 1,080 miles, and adding it to the radius of Earth, we get 5,040 miles, which again weaves the 108 and 54 threads through our phi reality. The pentagon, with its five 108-degree angles and 540-degree total, is the ultimate activator and container for all biology, and folding pentagonal faces into a ball creates the dodecahedron, which is at the core of DNA formation. Remember when I said that the Star Dodecahedron was a good choice for moving energy into the DNA molecule?

It has 10,800 degrees on its surface; and furthermore, it embodies the 12/60 numerical system we spoke about, with its 12 points and 60 faces. Also, 12 times 60 equals 720, which reflects a multiple of all of the platonic solids as well as the base angle (72°) of the phi ratio pyramids on the stellated dodecahedron. As mentioned earlier, this form resonates with the higher Christ body of consciousness, embodying compassion and heart-centered divine love.

Time has also been shown to be a three-dimensional construct affected by these same mathematical laws of creation. A number of authors and scientists have demonstrated a correlation between celestial movements and major Earth transformative events, especially concerning the cyclical nature of history. The key time period used is one fourth of an astrological age, which equals 540 years minus 1 year, to align with 11-year sun cycles.

All of these correlations demonstrate that the universe is resonant in both space and time *with the elemental angles and patterns* that are found within the pentagon and are reflections of life. Or is life an expected, unavoidable consequence of the universal rhythms of our space/time reality? Human beings have developed similar patterns that keep them close to the heartbeat of creation. A sincere soul realizes that a sequence of 108 prayers creates a resonant platform capable of delivering results consistent with the underlying truth of the universe and 107 misses the mark. However, many religions and spiritual practices still dance around the doorway, for without the proper understanding and use of 108, walking through the door is only a hope based on faith rather than an understanding based on experience.

FRED: So fascinating to see these spiritual and geometric relationships related to 108! What form do you feel is most powerful for pineal gland activation/Third Eye opening?

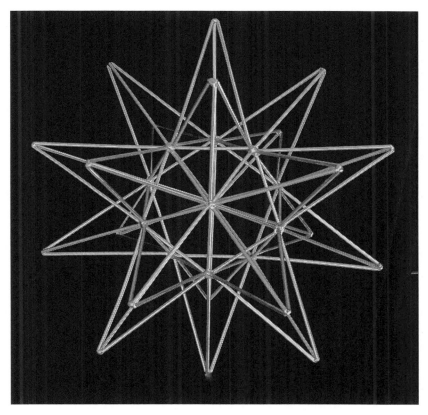

Star Icosahedron form by Greg Hoag

GREGORY: The phi Stellated (or Star) Icosahedron (above) *vibrates at a sixth-dimensional light-body level* and thus works well for pineal activation. Because it is intimately connected to the Stellated (Star) Dodecahedron (see page 119), it also has 10,800 degrees of angles on its surface. As the 20-sided platonic solid, it is the dual of the 12-sided dodecahedron (meaning one can be generated within the other). They dance back and forth through eternity via the phi ratio. The Unity Grid that I've created (see below) blends the dodecahedron and the icosahedron into a unique form, which resonates very high in the dimensional realms to also activate the Third Eye and create a unification of higher and lower consciousness, creating also a strong flow of energy between the heart and the head. The understanding here is that the heart is the doorway to the higher-dimensional realms and thus opens the pathway for higher self to interact with the physical brain. The Unity Grid is the third geometry to contain 10,800° and each of its sixty triangular faces is an exact duplicate of the faces on the Great Pyramid at Giza. The Rigveda, one of the oldest Sanskrit texts in the world, is made up of 10,800 stanzas, which is also the number of kiln-fired bricks in the Indian fire altar ritual (Agnicayana). Again, we are witnessing not coincidence, but a description of a divine gateway that can be constructed in our world for the purpose of spiritual evolution. Translating the encoded numbers into degrees gives us our answer.

FRED: I love the Unity Grid form, and as you know, I've placed two Unity Grids deep in the waters of Lake Titicaca Bolivia. One, I dropped in myself, to the north of Island of the Sun; the other I had placed by my friend Terry Smith, between the Islands of the Sun and Moon. These were placed to help reactivate the Divine Feminine energies of Gaia. The third was placed in a group sacred ceremony I participated in, with the help of a local Rapa Nui shaman at Easter Island in 2019. The intent of the latter is to reactivate ancient energies of Rapa Nui, healing this isolated island and its natives, and for it to then radiate this powerful geometric and crystalline energy like a beacon to help balance the rest of Gaia.

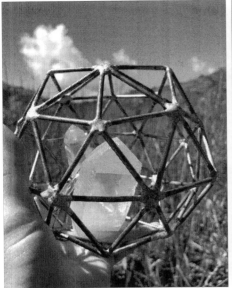
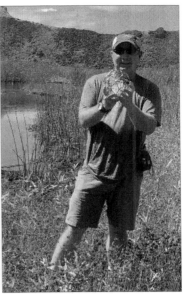

Unity Grid custom-made by Greg with author's Lemurian crystals inside

Author with Unity Grid (with enclosed Lemurian crystals) at Easter Island

Gregory, last but not least, the torus! How can we apply toroidal energy to our field to enhance our DNA and chakra balancing?

GREGORY: From the galaxies to our planet, from our whole body to each individual atom in our body, the way energy moves is through the shape of a torus. This is the energetic model for the way our third-dimensional reality is supported by the higher-dimensional levels. This is also seen in the energy flow of the chakras, nadis, and meridian system of the physical body.

All of the angular forms that we have already discussed are working with these unseen toroidal energies. We always work with a torus when we work with energy flow, as it stabilizes physical form and is the underlying energy matrix defining the spiral flow of the electromagnetic spectrum. It does this by creating a clockwise and counterclockwise spin in each of the axes (X-Y-Z) of 3-D reality simultaneously, for a total of 6 different simultaneous counter-rotating spins. This is why a smoke ring holds its shape in spite of the fact that it appears to be made of nothing. From its originating pulse, it moves outward around a core similar to a tornado or whirlpool spin that is reflexive and regenerating. It is also another demonstration of the nature of 6 being the underlying formative function of matter. A form as simple as a cube draws upon 13 interlinked toroids for its creation and energy flow. They are discovered through the total of its edges (12), vertices (8), and faces (6) divided by 2. For a toroid serves the yin/yang of every pair with the influx (North Magnetic Pole-black hole) and outflow (South Magnetic Pole-white hole).

So toroids represent the energetic aspect of everything in the physical dimension; however, I still use specific toroidal-shaped materials for energy flow in the chambers and jewelry forms.

Each jewelry piece is toroidal shaped with two openings, so they are directional in their energy flows—creating a grounding flow of energy or higher mental-energy flow, depending on its orientation to the body. Almost everything I create is a reflection of higher guidance, and my understanding of how and why it works is a case of reverse engineering what I've watched being made through me.

One of the more involved creations was a double torus constructed of geopolymers, which is similar to what people have done with mixing quartz and metal materials in a plastic resin. I don't care for most plastics, as they are amorphous, with no internal structure—thus blocking or deadening in nature. I used materials that were more like actual crystalline rock structure, formed with a high level of heat released during the process. Two toroids were stacked 2 inches apart, to form an 8-inch cube, and they were then infinity wrapped with vinyl tubing that had special materials pumped through. This was one component of a larger Toroidal Earth energizer that is programmed to run for twenty-four hours and then be off for seventy-two indefinitely, to impart energy into the Earth environment for healing and growth of both the planet and human beings. To heal the Mother is to heal ourselves.

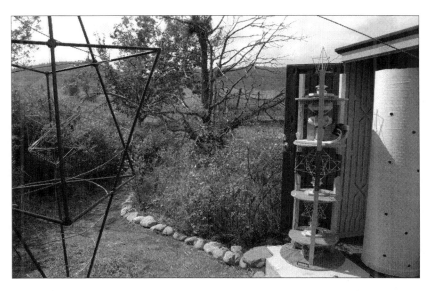

Toroidal Earth energizer on Greg's property near Lyons, Colorado

FRED: That's a very impressive toroidal field that it generates, and it's fascinating to hear that its programming and intention aim at healing the Earth and ourselves. My favorite use of toroidal flow is during my compassion meditations for the planet and its inhabitants. I visualize a full-spectrum light flowing down through the center of my heart, then circulate it back up around the outer heart, creating a toroid flow that eventually expands to my entire body and beyond. Guiding patients and friends in this meditative technique has been very powerful as well.

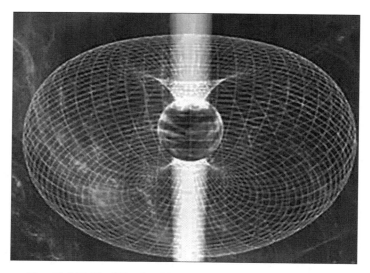

Toroidal Field of Earth—Nassim Haramein Facebook page

FRED: Thank you, Gregory, for your time and sacred-geometry insights that extend beyond our 3-D perceptions! Yes, I agree, we must respect and heal our planet if we are to heal ourselves. Digesting your content may take time for many of us, but you are seeding us with information that can be understood over time, allowing us to grasp even more complex geometries and relationships moving forward.

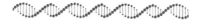

As Nassim Haramein, father of a fractal-holographic theory of the universe, tells us, "You are the surface on which the universe encodes information . . . you give the universe the surface to grow and learn."[109]

To summarize, sacred geometries found in nature and art can help harmonize our minds and bodies, as they are mirrored in our body—from DNA to the brain's neural networks and visibly in the curvatures in the human body. Appreciating these geometries as we hike or meditate in nature, whether observing the underside of a mushroom, a flower, a fern tendril, or the fractalization of branches in a tree, will nourish our soul and activate our healing DNA. Holding these geometric forms during meditation, wearing them, or experiencing expansive sacred geometry while being present in cathedrals, temples, and circles is also enlightening. As these observations force us to slow down, be present, and relax, our stress hormones decrease and further amplify the benefits as they turn off the inflammatory switches on your DNA.

Chapter 5
Sound: Creator and Healer

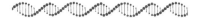

Music has touched the human soul across all
boundaries of time, space, and genre . . . Perhaps,
in its vibratory nature, music opens us to a greater
appreciation of our essential connectedness to the
cosmos, our oneness with all that is.

—Balfour M. Mount, urologic-cancer surgeon and
the Eric M. Flanders Emeritus Professor of
Palliative Care at McGill University

The effect of sound is more complex, multidimensional, and influential to life than can be comprehended by even the greatest scientific minds. As mathematicians, theoretical physicists, astrophysicists, acoustic scientists, and healers continue their passionate pursuit—analyzing sound at the quantum, local, and cosmic level with the aid of supercomputers—we will begin to piece this intricate puzzle together.

Ancient belief in the idea that sound played a major role in creation is found in a number of religious texts. For example, John

1:1, the King James version, reads: "In the beginning was the Word, and the Word was with God, and the Word was God." Similarly, in the Hindu Vedas: "In the beginning was Brahman with whom was the Word, and the Word is Brahman." An excerpt from *God Talks with Arjuna: The Bhagavad Gita by Paramahansa Yogananda* reads: "In point of fact, none can escape a constant communion with Aum, for it pervades the consciousness and every fiber and atom of every being. Those who become consciously attuned to the omnipresent Cosmic Vibration receive untold blessings."[110] ("The word" represents sound as vibration.)

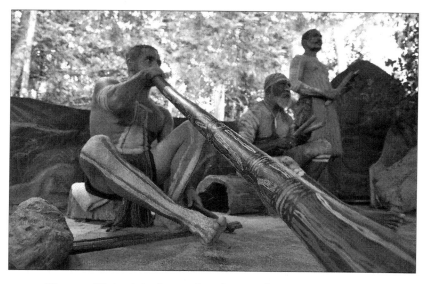

Yirrganydji aboriginal men play aboriginal music on didgeridoo and wooden instrument during aboriginal culture show in Queensland, Australia. Photo by ChameleonsEye (Shutterstock).

Historically speaking, the Australian aborigines were the earliest-known sound healers, their use of the didjeridu going back an estimated forty thousand years. They still use this long tube, often of hardwoods, hollowed out by insects such as termites. One can only wonder about the multitude of roles—from shamanic dreamwork and ceremonies in the Outback to the more modern uses in the developed world—the didjeridu has played over this time span. Two prominent researchers in this field note that these aborigines "healed broken bones, muscle tears, and illnesses of every kind using their enigmatic musical instrument," the yidaki (ancient name of the didjeridu).[111]

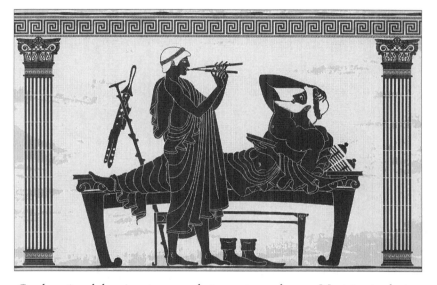

Greek national drawing: two men between two columns. Musician is playing on the pipe and the poet listens to him, by Hoika Mikhail (Shutterstock)

Beyond for entertainment, other ancient civilizations have used sound and music for deep healing. These include the Egyptians, the Greeks in the Pythagorean Mystery School, and the Maya in Mexico. Singing bowls forged by hammering a mix of metals date back 5,000 years to Mesopotamia, and later, during the time of Buddha 2,400 years ago, became prominent amongst Tibetan monks and shamans.

On a recent trip to the pre-Columbian city of Chichen Itza, I witnessed how the Maya aligned their pyramids not only to the stars and the equinoxes, but also acoustically designed them in one case to mimic the sound of a bird and serpent. For example, if you clap your hands at the base of the Kukulkan step pyramid (aka El Castillo), the echo is an ascending/descending birdlike chirp, reminiscent of the ascent/descent of the sacred quetzal Plumed Serpent (Kukulkan). The reverberating echo off a distant temple mimics a snake's rattle. Is this coincidence? It may well have been laid out by this highly sophisticated culture to represent the Feathered Serpent, Kukulkan, the temple honors. During the spring and fall equinox, thousands come to observe the shadow of a serpent descend down the pyramid, out the serpent mouth at the base, followed by the snake shadow slithering across the field in front of the pyramid. I truly doubt that the acoustic effects at Chichen Itza are coincidence.

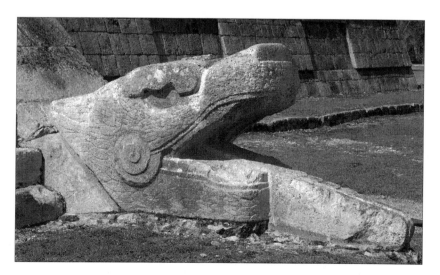

Kukulkan Serpent Head at the Base of El Castillo, Chichen Itza

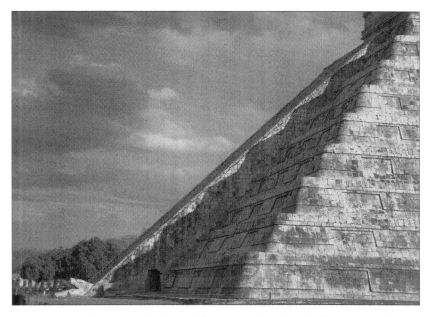

The Wavy Shadow of the Quetzalcoatl (Kukulkan)
serpent descending on the Equinox

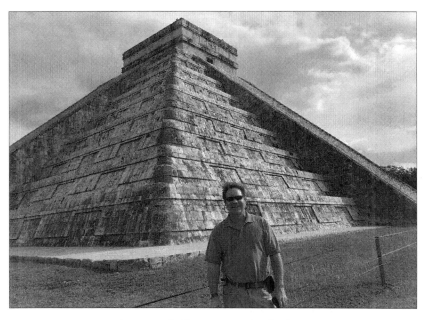

Author at Kukulkan Pyramid, Chichen Itza

Iamblichus' Life of Pythagoras, by Thomas Taylor, noted: "Pythagoras [c. 570–500 BC] considered that music contributed greatly to health, if used in the right way. He called his method 'musical medicine.' . . . To the accompaniment of Pythagoras his followers would sing in unison certain chants . . . At other times his disciples employed music as medicine, with certain melodies composed to cure the passions of the psyche . . . anger and aggression."[112] A statement by Demetrius, identified as "a Greek traveler," circa 200 B.C., describes the ritualistic use of sound: "In Egypt, when priests sing hymns to the Gods they sing the seven vowels in due succession and the sound has such euphony that men listen to it instead of the flute and the lyre."[113]

Modern-day sound healer/musician Jonathan Goldman, director of the Sound Healers Association, created this simple formula: Frequency (the actual sound used) + Intent (consciousness) = Healing.

He feels that when healthy, a person has a wonderful harmonic orchestra; it can become imbalanced if, by analogy, a violinist loses the sheet music and is out of rhythm. But if, as a conductor or sound healer, we can project the correct resonate frequency, we help vibrate that person back to health.[114] I am grateful to Jonathan and other masters for rebirthing much of the wisdom of the ancients, adding depth. Aided by their research, my own natural embrace of sound healing has allowed me to integrate it comprehensively in my medical practice. Recently, on Valentine's Day, I chanted with nearly a hundred people in sacred circle as part of Jonathan's World Sound Healing Day while thousands of people around the globe spent five minutes sounding "Ah" with the intent to send love to Mother Earth. It reminded me of why monks and all of us can receive precious gifts from our voices.

Cymatics, the study of sound in visible form, has become increasingly popular in recent years. For example, British acoustic-physics researcher John Stuart Reid pointed out, "Cymatics has captured the imagination of many thousands of people worldwide, perhaps because there is something almost magical about seeing matter move under the influence of sound."[115] The word "cymatics" was coined in the 1960s by Swiss medical doctor Hans Jenny (1904–'72), from the Greek *kyma*, meaning "wave." Jenny experimented mainly with particulate matter, such as sand and lycopodium powder vibrating on metal plates, and he published two lavishly illustrated volumes of his work. Inspired by Jenny, Reid conducted a cymatic experiment in Egypt's Great Pyramid in 1997, in which he stretched a plastic membrane across the open top of the sarcophagus, the 3.7 ton granite box in the King's Chamber. During the experiment, while sound throbbed throughout the chamber and its sarcophagus, he witnessed what appeared to be ancient Egyptian hieroglyphs manifesting in the sand he had sprinkled on the membrane, suggesting the possibility that cymatics could become a powerful new tool for science. Seeing hieroglyphic-like images form on the membrane seemed miraculous to Reid, but around twenty minutes into the experiment, he noticed that his painful lower-back condition (due to an injury sustained three weeks earlier) was also miraculously healed. This aspect of the experiment inspired his journey of exploration into the biological mechanisms that underpin sound therapy, which continues to this day.

In the years that followed his King's Chamber research Reid invented the CymaScope instrument, which imprints sonic vibrations on ultra pure water. Reid explained, "When sound encounters a membrane such as your skin or the surface of water, it imprints an invisible pattern of energy. In other words, the periodic vibrations in the sound sample are transposed to become periodic water ripples, creating beautiful geometric patterns that reveal the once hidden realm of sound."[116] Researchers worldwide now use this tool to make sound visible. Reid coined the word "CymaGlyph" to mean "sound image."[117]

At a recent conference, Reid detailed how these CymaGlyph patterns imprint "on the trillions of water-rich cellular membranes that make up the body. This interaction of sound on cellular membranes has triggered the emergence of sound as a powerful healing modality."[118]

Within a few milliseconds the water translates the large amount of sinusoidal (wavelike) information in a sound, resulting in a dynamic visible image in the water.

Similar to the discoveries following upon the introduction of the microscope or telescope, the CymaScope is helping researchers understand how—in fields as diverse as biology, astrophysics, and oceanography—our world and universe is influenced by sound. I have the CymaScope app on my iPhone, which, although comparatively low tech, gives me as I tone my crystal or Tibetan healing bowls a related geometric image. It's also a great teaching aid prior to a sound-therapy session with a patient.

The biology-research section of Reid's website, in "Cymatics—The Trigger for Life," hypothesizes that sound aided in the creation of life from the primordial soup of our oceans; i.e., that it helped amino acids, proteins, and other building blocks coalesce and organize: "What force was at work to cause the building blocks to coalesce, and begin to create form from formlessness?

We believe, just as the ancient seers prophesied, that the creative force was the most obvious and potent of all: sound. When sound interacts with matter cymatic forces organise the matter into microscopic and macroscopic structures." Again, this correlates well with John 1:1, "In the beginning was the Word."[119]

In the CymaGlyphs captured in their lab, "morphologies spontaneously and frequently appear that are reminiscent of early life." In the CymaScope laboratory, sound frequencies have re-created the morphologies of trilobites, starfish, diatoms, and radiolaria, to name a few early life forms. Are these images coincidence? he asks. Or are they an indication of a fundamental organizing principle?

The human voice can also be captured by the CymaScope instrument, beautifully demonstrated in the CymaGlyph titled "Reiki Chant." Reid commented, "We were asked by our friend and colleague Jonathan Goldman to image part of his *Reiki Chants* album, in which the harmony of voices is simply glorious to experience. When such sonic beauty imprints on water, the result is harmony within the water, not only on the surface but also at depth. In other words, the sound has organized the molecules throughout the body of the water. The "Reiki Chant" CymaGlyph shows this effect very well, with several layers of organization, but it has another noteworthy feature: its sevenfold form. Sevenfold cymatic forms are quite rare, and for a reason that my colleagues and I have not yet been able to explain, both men and women involved in spiritual practices, as is the case for Jonathan Goldman, typically create sevenfold CymaGlyphs. Whatever the reason for this, the fact that sonic beauty harmonizes water leads us to consider what happens in the human body when we are immersed in a beautiful soundscape? And conversely, how do our cells respond when we are immersed in a dissonant or noisy environment? Since our bodies are almost entirely comprised of water, these are important questions. My recent research is focused on finding answers, particularly at the cellular level."[120]

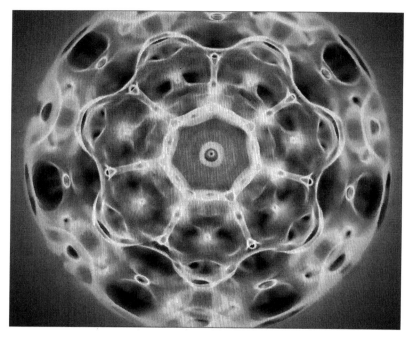

"Reiki Chant" CymaGlyph by John Stuart Reid

Reid speculates that hot gases from underwater hydrothermal vents create sounds that provided the organizing principle by which life emerged three billion years ago in Earth's primordial oceans. All pure (sinusoidal) sounds contain the all-important phi ratio; this creates "sonic scaffolding" that, he believes, organized, structured, and triggered life. In sum:

> We suggest the creative power of sound triggered
> life and continued to shape it, a process that is prob-

ably just as much at work today as it was in the primordial oceans and the early eras.

The shape of life, we believe, **is sound**."[121]

If sound was involved in the morphogenesis of life, does it continue to shape our DNA, which contains the phi ratio in the double helix? Did this ongoing primal resonance over millions of years assist in the evolution of life forms that eventually branched to us? Perhaps the alchemy of Earth sound frequencies, light, gravity, electromagnetism, and planetary cycles has helped organize simple and complex life forms into biorhythmic patterns too. An example of this is the precise timing of coral spawning each year.

Dr. Susumu Ohno, a world-renowned geneticist from the Beckman Research Institute in California, who developed theories of genetic sex determination and evolution through gene duplication, offered insights. A classical music lover, he ascribed notes to each of the amino acids that make up the DNA code. Interestingly, he found that by transcribing the sound pattern of DNA from living things, he could create music! Elaborating in the journal *Immunogenetics* in 1986, he wrote: "The all-pervasive principle of repetitious recurrence governs not only coding sequence construction but also human endeavor in musical composition."

He noted that the DNA of a particular type of cancer had an uncanny similarity to Chopin's *Funeral March*!

Of course, entrepreneurs have created a company that can translate your genome into music. (See the website Your DNA Song Ltd.) At the time of this writing, you can have them create a symphonic version of your genome for $550, after having the raw data processed through https://23andme.com or https://Ancestry. com. Sorry, no rock 'n roll or jazz available, just classical.

So if our DNA can create a musical composition, what happens in reverse? Ongoing research shows that using frequency-based tones, music, chanting, or even humming, we can change our predominant beta brainwave pattern to meditative alpha and theta states. As monks and other meditators chant mantras, they often enter into advanced spiritual states. Since we know that high cortisol levels can result in brain atrophy, reducing the stress-related steroid hormone cortisol through the meditative effects of sound and music will be regenerative, as it stimulates the growth and preservation of neurons (neurotropic benefit) and supportive microglia cells.

Daniel J. Levitin, the James McGill professor emeritus of psychology and behavioral neuroscience at McGill University in Montreal, says, "We've found compelling evidence that musical interventions can play a healthcare role in settings ranging from operating rooms to family clinics." Levitin, a former music producer and the author of four # 1 best-selling books, including *This is Your Brain on Music* (2006), added, "The researchers found that listening to and playing music increase the body's production of the antibody immunoglobulin A and natural killer cells—the cells that attack invading viruses and boost the immune system's effectiveness. Music also reduces levels of cortisol.[122]

To take one more example, in "Music Reduces Pain Perception in Healthy Newborns," in 2018, Italian researchers reported on an experiment in which healthy, randomly chosen newborns who had to undergo a painful medical procedure were exposed to either the regular, soothing *Mozart's Sonata for Two Pianos in D Major*, K. 448, or Beethoven's *Moonlight Sonata*, contrasted with newborns in a similar situation exposed to no music. They reported that "infants who were exposed to the three music interventions displayed a significant reduction in heart rate and in pain perception and an increase in oxygen saturation, as compared to the control group, which showed less modifications on stress measurements after painful medical procedures." They added that further research was needed to develop guidelines "and include music as a part of evidence-based strategies to promote the outcome for neonates."[123]

To convey how sound has impacted my life, I've included two examples below.

On a volunteer medical trip to Nepal in 2000, I inaugurated the venture with a climb to the top of Mount Kala Patthar. My father and a few others from our team joined in. On a fall morning we made the dangerous flight from Kathmandu, landing nearly 9,500 feet above sea level on the very short runway at Lukla dubbed "the most dangerous airport in the world." Sir Edmund Hillary, the first to summit Everest, had this small strip built for a supplies shipment prior to summiting Everest with his Sherpa guide, Tenzing Norgay, in 1953. With the runway just under five hundred yards long, carved into the side of a mountain, a small miscalculation can mean smacking into the cliff at the end of the runway. The damaged planes off the side of the runway attest to this!

After a white-knuckled landing and some deep breaths we hired two hardy, elite Sherpas—Pemba and Perba—to assist in carrying our packs and guiding us to the summit. The Sherpas are ethnic Tibetans, many of whom migrated to Nepal when the Chinese took over Tibet in 1950. Our goal was to escape fast-approaching pressures and get a close-up, panoramic view of Everest, the mountain with the highest altitude in the world (29,035 feet above sea level), prior to setting up our large health camp in north-central Nepal in the dusty village of Barabise.

The Mount Kala Patthar trek is a sixty-miles round trip with frequent ups and downs in elevation, wild suspension-bridge crossings, and—to avoid being knocked off the trail—special attention given to passing yaks, goats, and large-load-carrying Sherpas. The summit, at 18,514 feet, has the best panoramic views of Everest, the nearby peaks, Khumbu Glacier, and the base camp below, reached via a safer, easier route. Did I contemplate climbing Everest? Yes, but after seeing the oversized egos of folks that had climbed it and trashed it, I decided I didn't want to become one of them. Besides, why spend over forty grand to have a 10 percent chance of dying from the Khumbu Glacier falling on me, or the numerous other potential risks such as losing brain cells from hypoxia. I need those to take me to ninety, at least!

As with most treks, the journey itself outweighs in importance the endpoint. By far the most significant experience en route occurred in tiny Tengboche—at an elevation of over 12,000 feet—about halfway to South Everest Base Camp. The village and its Buddhist monastery sit against the backdrop of mystical Ama Dablam mountain, with Everest in the distance.

We overnighted in a small lodge that looks down at this enigmatic monastery. The morning before we hit the trail, we joined the monks in prayer, even as Hillary and Tenzing had prior to beginning the ascent of Everest. Inside the large stone monastery,

162

the walls are filled with beautiful Buddhist paintings, and the ceilings with large hanging thangkas; at the altar there is a big gold-painted Buddha. We were invited to sit quietly in meditation with about twenty monks, who began a guttural chant, reciting the Om Mani Padme Hum mantra—repeated over and over. The deep rhythmical tones conducted through my muscles and bones shifted me into a mystical state as the mantra, which is said to contain all of the Buddha's teachings, sonically entranced my mind and body. Wikipedia explains: "Thus the six syllables, om mani padme hum, mean that in dependence on the practice of a path which is an indivisible union of method and wisdom, you can transform your impure body, speech, and mind into the pure exalted body, speech, and mind of a Buddha." As I closed my eyes, I felt a detachment from time. It seemed as though we were traveling in a different dimension with the monks, sensing oneness and compassion for the planet and its inhabitants.

Before long, a Tibetan tingsha (symbol) chime sounded, and I was out of my hypnotic state, back in reality, thinking of the conceivably deadly hike ahead. I felt relaxed, revived in a way I could not explain, wondering how it might affect me in the near and distant future. I wondered if untold numbers of monks, chanting together, had imprinted it with an intentional potency.

Sound healer Jonathan Goldman best captures what I was feeling:

> There are two main ways that sound affects us. The first is called "psycho-acoustics." These are sounds that go into our ears and into our brain, affecting our nervous system, including our heart rate and respiration. As noted, this can produce great therapeutic

benefits and is certainly something that occurs when we listen to music. The second is called "vibro-acoustics." These are sounds that go into our body and vibrate us on a cellular level. While all sound (including music) that we hear has some vibro-acoustic ability, there are some sounds that in particular are extremely non-musical, yet quite excellent on vibrating the physical body. Humming is, in fact, the most powerful self-created sound that we know of which can produce vibro-acoustic effects, enabling the sounds to internally massage us and affecting us in the way that no other such sound can do.[124]

More recently I found myself in a completely different situation in the middle of the Pacific Ocean. Seated comfortably in an Adirondack chair, with my toes sunk deep in the warm, volcanic sand, I was listening to traditional Hawaiian music. I contemplated my location and realized I was at the base of a volcano that—measured from the seafloor—is taller than Everest and surrounded by the world's largest ocean. Aware of my feet connecting to the base of this volcano on the ocean floor, whose field enlarges into the ocean, then feeling it extend up the slopes to the summit helped me appreciate the ancient Hawaiian's relationship with earth, fire, air, and water. Mauna Kea is merged with four other sacred volcanoes that make up the Big Island; it was created by the energies of Goddess Pele, according to Hawaiians, or by a geological hot spot per modern-day scientists.

As I enjoyed myself at a beach restaurant the sun began to set; trade winds lightly swayed the palm trees, and in the soft sand my bare feet became even more content. I basked in the company of twenty family members and caught up with my cousin Mike, a well-known island artist.

Two musicians playing Hawaiian music were soon accompanied by a hula dancer. The graceful flow of the dance synced perfectly with the swaying palms and the waves rolling onto the sandy beach.

Drawn from their tables, several young children began to dance in the sand in front of the dancer. In a matter of minutes, the kids connected to the drum rhythm and the flow of hula. These were not natives, but mainland kids, who had likely rarely heard Hawaiian music.

I knew there had to be something akin to animal instinct that allowed them to drop into the genre so quickly. Parents joined in, but couldn't spontaneously connect into the natural flow. Witnessing children dancing to rock at wedding receptions and other celebrations never seemed to phase me, but watching them quickly align to the hula flow intrigued me.

As I reflected on this, it became obvious that children were sonically entraining their brains and movement to the music better than their parents.

Could it be that their less developed, less scrutinizing frontal cortex was allowing the music to resonate and flow more freely to their deep brain structures, motor cortex, and cerebellum associated with movement? I'd hypothesize that children perceive sound in a more energetically connected, kinesthetic way than adults, whose thickened cortex impedes and filters the flow.

In this regard, many mothers are now playing music to their fetus in the second and third trimesters in hopes of creating smarter, less anxious children. Alfred A. Tomatis, a French ENT (Ear, Nose, Throat) physician, determined that fetuses can hear in utero at approximately four and a half months.[125] Considered the Einstein of the ear, he developed an Electronic Ear, which has effectively stimulated and balanced neural pathways to address learning disabilities and emotional disturbances. His Tomatis Method deploys sound therapy to enhance motor, emotional, and cognitive abilities.[126] He and Robert Monroe, founder of the Monroe Institute, researched the phenomenon of sonic entrainment, where certain sound frequencies, sometimes varied from one ear to the other, can make the brain synchronize into a specific brainwave pattern, such as beta or theta. Monroe's Hemi-Sync® patented audio technology created binaural beats that—depending on the tracks played—can shift someone into relaxation, enhanced learning, or an altered state of consciousness.[127]

Explaining why sound and music so strongly affect us, Andrew Weil, MD, focused on entrainment, noting that "various bodily processes—respiration, heart rate, and brainwaves—synchronize with the frequencies of what we hear and feel. For example, a stroll along the beach becomes deeply relaxing as body rhythms entrain to the lulling sound of ocean waves. When you listen to slow, relaxing music, your heart naturally beats more slowly, breathing deepens, and brain waves slow down—all of which are linked with relaxation and healing."[128]

What if sound therapy could reduce the incidence of Cesarean sections?

Ron Minson, MD, Clinical Director of Integrated Listening Systems (iLs), has been using sound therapy since 1990 to help children and adults overcome struggles with attention, learning, behavior, and mood disorders. Not long ago, in conversation with me, he shared information about a most unique and relatively unknown use of sound: in therapy for pregnant mothers. From his close relationship and training with Tomatis, Dr. Minson explained:

> Dr. Tomatis was telling a number of us about a research study with pregnant mothers in two separate Paris hospitals. By this time, Tomatis was delivering his sound-therapy program through special headphones that transmitted Mozart's music and Gregorian chants through both air and bone conduction. (A bone conductor—a large hearing aid—inserted into the headphone band, sends gentle vibrations of sound through the skeletal system.)
>
> For five days, during the fifth and the eighth months of gestation, pregnant women listened to the music. The outcome showed a statistically significant decrease in the use of anesthetics, a decrease in episiotomies, and a marked decrease in Caesarean sections.
>
> I clearly understood how there could be a decreased use of anesthetics and fewer episiotomies as a result of the proven effects of sound therapy in decreasing stress and anxiety, thus relaxing the mother and pelvic floor. I was most excited about how this approach could also decrease Cesarean section rates.
>
> Dr. Tomatis explained, "The primary reason for Cesarean sections is a breech (butt first) presentation. The sound and vibration of the music is carried from

the skull along the spinal column into the pelvis. The unborn infant will turn itself to a head-down position, placing its head in the pelvis to better receive the nurturing music and, of course, the mother's voice."

Dr. Minson went on:

> I loved using sound therapy with pregnant mothers and in 2001 added a pregnancy program into the training of therapists. In 2007, it was incorporated into the extensive iLs repertoire of therapy programs now used by over 8,000 trained educators and therapists worldwide. Currently, from the fifth month of pregnancy, mothers-to-be may listen as much as they wish.
>
> I continue to receive reports from excited mothers whose babies inverted *spontaneously* during the pregnancy program. Recently, an iLs occupational therapist called to tell me that during the first hour of listening, her baby turned spontaneously. She'd been scheduled to have an external version by her obstetrician the following day, but avoided this painful and risky procedure, thanks to the sound therapy leading her baby into a vertex, head-down position. An external version involves the obstetrician using their hands on a mother's belly to push and rotate the infant to a head-down position (going from breech to vertex) in the pelvis. Sometimes the cord can be compressed, or the placenta can be injured while performing this, leading to a C-section and other serious complications for mother and infant. (For more information on iLs, www.integratedlistening.com)

Through the early work of Tomatis and Monroe, furthered by advancements by Jonathan Goldman, Barry Goldstein, Kimba Arem, Tom Kenyon, Peter Kater, Robert Coxon, and many other sound healers, we are fine-tuning the application of frequency and harmony with compassionate intent, to heal and balance our spiritual, emotional, mental, and physical bodies. I have also found mantra music to be open my heart, third, and crown chakra in ways I never would have imagined. The mantras sung with musical accompaniment by my favorite artists, such as Snatam Kaur, Ajeet Kaur, Krishna Das, Deva Primal, Guru Ganesha, Donna De Lory, and Mirabai Ceiba, offer a powerful means to meditate deeply or enjoy on a hike in nature. Regarding classical music, a 1993 study (Rauscher et al.) showed an improvement in spatial IQ while listening to a Mozart sonata for just ten minutes.[129] This was the so-called Mozart effect, a term coined two years earlier by Alfred Tomatis—author of *Pourquoi Mozart? (Why Mozart?)*.

Returning a year later to build on their 1993 study, the University of California Irvine researchers Frances H. Rauscher et al. delivered a follow-up in 1994 at the American Psychological Association 102nd Annual Convention, in Los Angeles:

> The second experiment, presented at the meeting by Dr. Rauscher and Dr. Shaw, expanded on their widely reported study published by *Nature* in October 1993, which found that listening to 10 minutes of Mozart's Piano Sonata K 448 increased spatial IQ scores in college students, relative to silence or relaxation instructions. The new findings replicated the effect, and found no increase in spatial skills after subjects listened to 10 minutes of either a composition by Philip

Glass or a highly rhythmic dance piece, suggesting that hypnotic musical structures will not enhance spatial skills. Dr. Rauscher and Dr. Shaw suggest that these two complementary studies have serious educational and scientific implications. "We are in the process of designing further studies directed toward strengthening the enhancing effect of music training on spatial reasoning that we found for the preschoolers. We hope our research will help convince public school administrators of how crucial music instruction is to all children," they explained. Dr. Rauscher and Dr. Shaw also plan experiments to examine the neuronal mechanisms responsible for the causal link between music and spatial intelligence.[130]

Recently, while attending a summer concert by the famous cellist Yo-Yo Ma at Red Rocks Amphitheater west of my Denver home, I pondered the controversies surrounding the "Mozart effect" presented by Rausher, Shaw, and others. Attending concerts at this National Historic Landmark, regardless of music genre, is something everyone should experience in their lifetime!

As he played Bach cello suites eloquently and flawlessly on the barren stage, my mind began to let the visual-spatial stimulations sink in. No light show or dancers: just him—and a silent crowd tapping into his vibrating strings, stroked masterfully with the bow though the flow of his masterful brain and his collective consciousness into his arms and hands. Sitting in a place where Jurassic dinosaurs once roamed and surrounded by this naturally shaped sandstone amphitheater—watching Yo-Yo play from memory two hours straight, with the occasional bow or sip of water—was impressive. What struck me the most that summer eve was the sequential memory needed to play all these cello suites!

I had the insight that perhaps simply listening to classical music was not enough to enhance our brains, but learning to play the instrument and sequencing movements of a suite, sonata, or symphony was the missing link to embed neural tracts and create lasting cognitive enhancements of the "Mozart effect." Passive listening while having my cup of coffee in the morning definitely stimulates my visual spatial cortex and more. But an enduring competency would likely require an extra step: to pick up a cello or violin or sit down at the piano, for instance. Granted, a young child who inherited a brain primed for music may be shifted more profoundly than others, including myself.

At home I looked to see if anyone had researched sequencing and located a 2017 study in the journal *Psychology of Music* that confirmed this. It reported that although between musicians and non-musicians, "no differences were found in visual-spatial implicit statistical learning . . . robust differences were found in overall visual-spatial sequence learning abilities. Musicians displayed enhanced visual-spatial sequence learning and they consistently outperformed non-musicians in both phases of the Visual-Spatial Sequence Learning Task."[131]

After reviewing the studies, I believe that simply listening to classical is not enough. Again, if to epigenetically shift our DNA and build the neural tracts in our cortex, perhaps learning to play an instrument is needed. Further studies should shed more light on this hypothesis.

And it will be interesting to see whether listening to music or tones in a "sound lounger" (that vibrates through the body almost as if one were lying on a cello) would stimulate these tracts without the need to pick up an instrument. A deeper immersion beyond our headphones and surround sound is needed for enhanced entrainment, in my opinion. Feeling it inside, or being a part of it, is the missing element.

I asked my friend Suzannah Long, cofounder of So Sound® Solutions, her thoughts on the topic. Her cofounder, Barry Oser, designed So SoundHearts®, an advanced toroidal-shaped speaker that can be installed in a massage-therapy table, mattress, custom sound lounger, hospital bed, and even on a yoga floor. Anything from aboriginal didjeridu to ZZ Top via an MP3 player can be run through it. She elaborates:

> Listening to sound and music through your ears provides one level of experience. Feeling it resonate through your entire body/mind simultaneously, like a musical massage, quite literally amplifies the experience exponentially. . . . So as you relax upon a lounger, bed, floor, treatment table, etc., that is specially designed to deliver the sound and music tactilely, you naturally support a sensory integration experience that promotes deep relaxation and a sense of inner peace or body/mind harmonization. It also makes sense that as we expose the cells of our body to music, they would respond like water on a CymaScope plate. Our clients consistently share that they feel it is improving circulation, reducing pain, supporting enhanced creativity, mental clarity/coherence. And we are able to see from working with

bio- and neurofeedback devices in nonclinical research that through our acoustic-resonance technology, we are helping users balance heart rate, blood
pressure, brainwave states, and more.

Another case in point is "listening through the feet." As Jonathan
Goldman reminded me, "cymatherapy is a potential aspect of
sound therapy that represents the medicine of the future. Based
on the work of Dr. Peter Guy Manners, MD, it is of course, . . .
controversial." Among other instruments, Dr. Manners uses the
AMI™ 750, an Acoustic Meridian intelligence device designed by
Mandara Cromwell, described on the Cyma Technologies website as "based on the effectiveness of acoustic sound traveling the
energy pathways of the meridian system to relax and support the
body's balance." To use it, "Sit in a comfortable chair and relax your feet on supportive gel pads while the body uptakes the
sound frequencies through the feet."

Does it work? Impressively, yes, as evidenced in "Case Study:
the Efficacy of Equine Cymatechnologies Bioresonance on a
Superficial Digital Flexor Tendon Core Lesion of a Thoroughbred
Racehorse Colt." In the twenty-seventh annual meeting of
Bioelectromagnetics Society (BEMS) in Dublin in 2005, Dr.
Anthony Fleming "presented findings of an acoustic therapy device, the Cyma 1000, successfully trialed on thoroughbred racehorses. The work presents the photon and the phonon as two
particles having the same structure, but a different propagation
vector. The phonon is orthogonal to the photon of equivalent
energy. The phonon has the important advantage of being able
to penetrate far deeper into biological tissues than EM radiation.
Delivery of precise frequencies enable control over the DNA

bases during replication. This can be used to promote healing within injured tissues. The method is a generic process for a number of different important therapies." In conclusion, in this case "Equine cymatechnologies Bioresonance treatments have surpassed any standard veterinary treatment of the SDFT [superficial digital flexor tendon] injured horse by approximately 5 to 22.5 months ahead of any known standard treatments provided in the literature."[132]

From numerous sound healers I've spoken with, the general consensus is that resonating sound *through* your body, and not just your ears, taking it further than simply listening, transmutes a deeper intelligence, energy, and neurological entrainment.

If we want to *sense* the sound of waves, I recommend jumping in and feeling the kinetic energy, bringing in those extra-dimensional inputs through our body! My most memorable personal experience that documents this occurred while scuba diving deep in the Pacific off Maui, where I could feel and hear the eerie songs of humpback whale.

In my office I do my best to create a multidimensional experience in our mind spa. I haven't been able to create the *Star Trek* holodeck yet or scuba diving with humpbacks, but I'm working on it! Transmitting healing sounds to both headphones as well as coherent vibration tones through a sound-integrated massage table, I then add in—from a boom about two feet above a patient's head—the PandoraStar flashing-light therapy. [133]

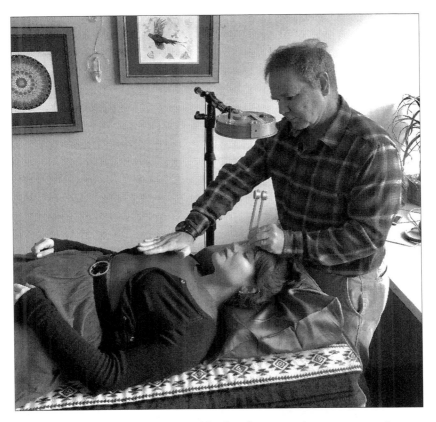

The author performing sound healing by resonating mantra music through the sound table, applying a tuning fork to the Third Eye, and doing energy work. The PandoraStar above her head can also be used, if desired, for even deeper work.

Using sound and light allows even my toughest Type A's (racing mentally through their to-do list) and ADD patients to drop rapidly into a deep meditative state. Periodically through the HeartMath program, which shows how well a person is remaining in a deep meditation, we assess their heart rate variability. Of course, I have a sound lounger at home to meditate on and rebalance my energy body with too!

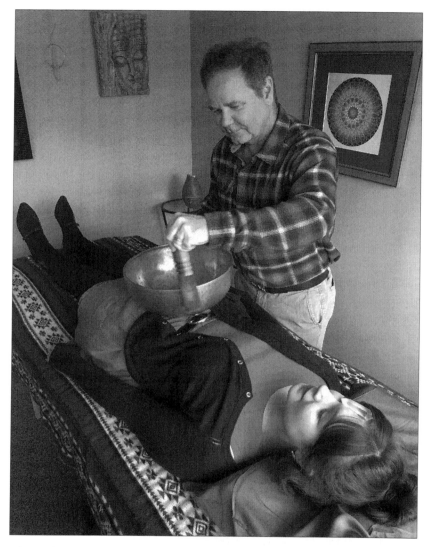

The author resonating his favorite Tibetan bowl in performing sound healing

When we move away from sympathetic drive (fight or flight/ stress) into parasympathetic (relaxed), a more varied (healthy) heart rate occurs. With this program, we can fine-tune the music on the massage-therapy table, resonating sound and the frequency and pattern of light. I also use Tibetan bowls, crystal healing bowls, and tuning forks.

I currently draw on seven types of healing in my sound-therapy/mind-spa room. At least three are used, and occasionally on longer sessions all of them. They include the following:

1. Singing bowls (crystal and Tibetan hammered alloy metal)

2. Tuning forks, weighted and unweighted

3. Sound table (massage table with special speakers, So SoundHearts by So- Sound Solutions, that transduce healing music from an iPod or CD player)

4. A Richway Amethyst BioMat, laid on top of the sound table (it has crystals woven into it, transmitting far-infrared heat for relaxation)

5. Near-infrared Pulsed LED light therapy pads by in-Light™ to apply as needed to areas of inflammation

6. Lemurian crystals to apply to chakras if desired by client

7. PandoraStar photic entrainment device

Each of these modalities may possess vibro-acoustic and/or psycho-acoustic healing effects. Which instrument to select is determined by the healing or balancing needed. Much of this comes out in the patient interview, but the rest is intuitive. In some ways, when I look around at all my instruments, I feel like I've created a sound-healing operating room!

I am fortunate to have the option of using quartz-crystal bowls or antique Tibetan hammered (multi-metal) singing bowls. The crystal bowls have a purer-toned clearing and energizing feel, whereas the metal bowls possess greater character and an inherent wisdom from over a century of use. Oftentimes, to do vibro-acoustic healing I reach for weighted or unweighted tuning forks rather than bowls. Weighted forks can work well to lightly complement sound-table therapy, fostering deeper states of relaxation and vibrating the Third Eye, as well as the sternum for the heart chakra as I gently apply them. Unweighted forks are tapped and then held around the head for auditory entrainment. This vibro-acoustic therapy helps open and connect the chakras. Energy work may also be performed in this setting if desired by the client.

In a treatment room adjacent to my mind spa, I have another massage table integrated with sound, which provides pulsed magnetic-field therapy (PEMFT). For those who aren't familiar with it, here's a description:

> Pulsed electromagnetic field therapy replicates the Earth's natural magnetic field, which we were once strongly connected to. Over time this magnetic field has gotten weaker (*an estimated 10% weaker since the 19th century*) and due to industrialization and modernization, we are further separated from the Earth's natural magnetic field. The therapy actually originated from NASA's research involving the benefits of pulsed electromagnetic fields on astronauts for fatigue, depression, bone loss and other symptoms

following even short trips to outer space. Scientists discovered that the cause was due to astronauts being without this beneficial natural field emanating from our Earth.[134]

Using this powerful device (known as the "Pulse"), we can pulse twenty teslas of magnetic wavelike energy (a tesla measures magnetic flux density) into a patient's entire body or specific regions of it to reduce inflammation, while at the same time resonating healing sounds through the massage table. Using these alchemies of light/sound/magnetism provides levels of healing not available even in large integrative medicine centers.

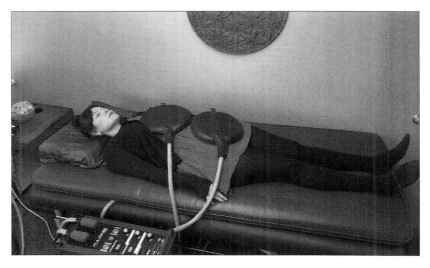

Pulse magnetic therapy to full body on the sound therapy table. An alchemy of sound and magnetic therapy.

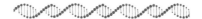

Looking for more answers, I sought out internationally recognized Boulder sound therapist, musician, and author Kimba Arem.[135] Her favorite tools include overtone-rich indigenous instruments such as the quartz-crystal didjeridu she designed, indigenous flutes, the waterphone, and Tibetan and crystal singing bowls. Naturally drawn to the didjeridu after a near-death experience in 1992, she found it transformed her life, as well as the many others she has since touched with it.

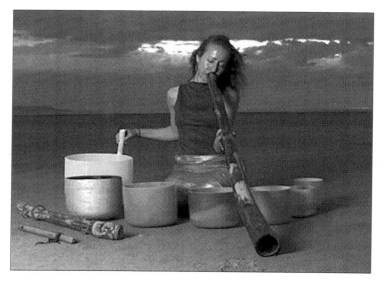

Kimba playing crystal bowl and didjeridu

FRED: How do you heal with sound?

KIMBA: When I'm playing an instrument, I'm actually intending to create a field of resonance to stimulate the individual to access their own healing ability.

She feels the didjeridu is an extension of the instrument of her body. As her hero, St. Francis of Assisi, said, "Make me an instrument of peace."

KIMBA: When I play the didjeridu, I feel connected to all of creation and can extend my breath/Spirit and intention through it to help others. I let the sound flow through me, through the circular breath, letting go of ego, and allow it to connect to unity consciousness . . . which I feel is part of the Gaian planetary supermind.

Like her dear friend and colleague Jonathan Goldman, she knows that having the right intention is key. Intentions involving status or monetary gain have no place in this benevolent field.

FRED: Do you feel an element of sonic entrainment occurs? (As a reminder, sonic entrainment is the ability of sound to stimulate the brain to enter a brainwave pattern such as predominately meditative theta state.)

KIMBA: Yes, through the vibration of sound, a field-like effect can be created and shared with others. Especially with the drone/OM-like sound of the didjeridu. Sound can be like a midwife, shifting brainwave patterns, restructuring the water in the body, and helping to facilitate major transformative processes, such as a shifting in consciousness, birthing, dying, or just letting go of old patterns and ways of being.

FRED: OK, so how does the geometry of sound heal?

KIMBA: Just as water can be structured by sound and energy, so can we. In the movie *Secret of Water* that I scored and coproduced,[136] Dr. Masaru Emoto [the pioneering researcher] demonstrated

. . . that water can be energetically enhanced as it flows down a mountain waterfall, but loses its symmetrical geometry as it flows through city pipes or is exposed to negativity and toxic elements. Sound with intentional healing frequencies can help water crystalize in more intricate, sacred geometric shapes. Water in the human body can be physically restructured by sound, providing another level of coherence and healing. Just as snowflakes all have unique shapes, each of us is also a unique vibratory being, so different sounds will affect each of us in unique ways.

FRED: Yes, I love Masaru's book and was impressed to see the beautiful images of water that came from natural sources and those from city or polluted water that were transformed through sound. It seems logical that a healing voice, singing bowls, the didjeridu, mantra music, classical music, etc., can be healing, but what about genres such as rock music?

KIMBA: Yes, some forms of rock music can be healing when there's positive intention and harmony. However, those that project rage, hatred, and disharmonious sounds may be harmful to health. Plants will grow in the opposite direction of speakers projecting such music. We can deduce that not all sound is symmetrical, coherent, geometrical, and harmonious.

An example of rock music with harmonious geometry is Sting's "Fragile," depicted growing beautiful geometrical crystals in a photo in Secret of Water. *Kimba feels that "when we hear harmony, we also feel it in our hearts. It's interesting that the word 'ear' is in the middle of the word heart. And is the first three letters in Earth."*

FRED: Current studies suggest that dolphin communication may be 3-D holographic in nature, and even *sono*graphic—allowing their fellow dolphins to see a fetus in a pregnant dolphin, for example. It was discovered in 2011 by Swedish and U.S. researchers that "dolphins and porpoises use echolocation for hunting and orientation . . . dolphins can generate two sound beam projections simultaneously." But a newer finding, in 2016, impresses me greatly:

> Recently scientists have made a significant breakthrough in inter-species communication. Researchers in the UK and USA have proved that the clicking sounds dolphins use for echolocation actually form reproducible holographic pictures that the researchers suggest may be the basis of dolphin language.[137]

The technology used to image echolocation pictures is the CymaScope instrument, which imprints dolphin sounds onto pure water, *rendering them visible*. This research is a collaboration between acoustic-physics researcher John Stuart Reid (UK) and dolphin researcher Jack Kassewitz (U.S.). In their groundbreaking experiments Kassewitz placed a series of plastic objects, such as a plant pot and cube, in the dolphin pool and tasked a dolphin to echolocate on each object. As the dolphin's echolocation beam reflected off each object a small portion of the beam, now modulated by the shape of the object, was picked up by a nearby hydrophone, a type of underwater microphone. The recorded hydrophone signal was sent to Reid's laboratory by email attachment. Astonishingly, when the echolocation signals were injected individually into the CymaScope, the shape of each object became visible in the water. After the success of this first series of experiments Kassewitz arranged for a full person (Jim McDonough) to be submerged in the pool, and the dolphin was tasked to echolocate on his face. But amazingly, when Reid imaged the file, the whole of McDonough was clearly visible.

The story of this breakthrough reverberated around the world, and a scientific paper was published in the *Journal of Marine Science*: "A Phenomenon Discovered While Imaging Dolphin Echolocation Sounds."[138] Subsequently, Kassewitz used 3-D printing technology to print a "what the dolphin saw" image of McDonough on plastic. The CymaScope images of dolphin sound pictures resemble early ultrasonography images, the technology used in hospitals to monitor a baby in the womb, in that they are monochrome and quite fuzzy. But Reid believes the technique can be developed to the point where sono-pictorial imagery approaching the resolution enjoyed by dolphins will eventually be possible. This amazing discovery has exciting implications for the future as the first step in being able to potentially communicate with dolphins in their own language.

KIMBA: Yes, they are producing and interpreting complex sound structures. Perhaps they have a more advanced, less atrophied pineal gland that gives them greater perception of these sound geometries as well. They also seem to be able to project sound healing to other beings in need, too.

FRED: Are there certain tonal values or notes that may balance chakras?

KIMBA: I don't think it is well established which notes affect various chakras. It's not as simple as that. Every individual likely resonates a chakra level with a unique note or tone, just as each of us has a unique vibratory frequency. We're all like pure white light that's been fractionated into the colors of the rainbow. In the third dimension we seem to have energy-body layers, such as emotional, mental, physical; or even the chakras seem to be separate colors/vibrations . . . and time seems to be linear as well. In the higher dimensions, these things are not perceived as separate colors or chakras or bodies . . . or even separate moments in time. But here in 3-D, we experience them as we do.

Just like the chakras, our organs and cells each have a unique resonate frequency. So, which sound goes with which chakra will be unique to the individual. Socrates said that if you study the monochord (a single note), you will discover the secrets of the universe. Therefore, any one single note can be directed anywhere in the body, and our intention can also help direct it where it needs to go . . .

KIMBA CONTINUED: Sound as medicine is infinitely complex . . . there are no masters . . . the mastery of the work is about showing up, being fully present in service to another, with a very thin ego membrane . . . and therefore being the messenger of the sound. Then the transfer of vibrational energy is pure. Essentially, it is about getting out of the way to let the sound do the work.

FRED: Perhaps our work is to synthesize our modern knowledge of sound healing, cymatics, and consciousness with that of the ancient Egyptians, Greeks, and others.

KIMBA: *Yes, consciousness is vibration, and when consciousness is structured into geometric patterns, it's coherent.* As we see in cymatics, one vibration causes a complex geometrical pattern. But as it starts to increase in frequency the geometrical pattern dissipates into chaos, until the next nodal point is reached and a new geometry emerges—more complex and coherent. Similarly, right now, it seems that our collective consciousness is shifting frequencies and we are "between geometries," so to speak. So the times seem quite chaotic. It is currently not coherent, because the new, more complex geometry of consciousness has not established itself. But as we continue to increase in frequency on the planet (and by the way, all of the planets in our solar system are "heating up," or increasing in frequency), we will soon see a new, more complex, harmonious geometry emerge.

FRED: Do you hope for a group consciousness that is coherent and trending towards a state of oneness?

KIMBA: Yes, I have seen for some time that the new level of co-herence on Gaia is the group-mind geometry collective, or unity consciousness. I have experienced moments of this a number of times in groups—and felt each time that these were previews of the next stage of humanity's evolution. Like bees, which operate as a collective organism in service to the planet, we too can link our consciousness in co-creative oneness. Bees create hexagonal shapes in their honeycomb, which is the same pattern in the heart field, and the geometry of water and space (as my friend [physicist] Nassim Haramein outlines in his work). They are displaying the Flower of Life geometry as a supermind.

FRED: Interesting. Perhaps humans can achieve supermind capabilities if they can connect to this group/universal consciousness to expand beyond the limit of our limited human brain. I feel the consciousness pot is being stirred, and many are beginning to resonate with the group-mind collective. Do you feel that sound therapy and healing may help catalyze coherency in humans?

KIMBA: Yes . . . and since my near-death experience in 1992, I have been directed as my life's calling to use sound and vibration as tools to help create group geometry and enable us to reach more-coherent states.

FRED: I'm concerned about the recent major drop in our bee population, perhaps related to incoherent (to us) wireless noise from cell-phone towers, which includes UHF, or ultra-high frequency (microwave), as well as to global warming, viral threats, mites. And last, but not least, pesticides. My family bee hive has taken some hits, but we are doing all we can to keep them healthy. This wireless noise alone must be affecting all living organisms in our ecosystem, making it more difficult to become coherent. What's your opinion on how harmful wireless noise is?

KIMBA: Well, it is worrisome. Our biology perhaps hasn't evolved to the point of adapting to the onslaught of the new frequencies being introduced at this time. But the more we can connect and ground into the field of our planet, such as walking barefoot in nature, meditating, etc., the better we can maintain biological coherence. *We are electrical beings, and if we do not allow ourselves to discharge the static (oxidation) that builds up in our systems, we get out of balance.* We here on Earth are on our planetary spaceship, our mother Gaia, and she is on a journey of transformation. If we want to go on this evolutionary journey with her and if we are not connected to the web of symbiotic life here, disharmony may arise.

FRED: Perhaps a combination of mindfulness, sound, spirituality, immersion in nature, and other strategies will keep us on the path.

In regard to energy fields, Princeton University's Global Consciousness Project has been hard at work connecting the dots. Monitoring international sites, they study the randomness or structured order (coherence) of collective emotion in highly charged events (such as the inauguration of President Barack Obama). The repeated finding is that charged collective emotion slightly *but significantly* derandomizes the random number generators (RNGs) measuring the response at locations around the world. HeartMath Institute commented: "So far we have taken an exploratory look at the possibility of global events being the catalyst for the kind of coherence that we think of as a global consciousness."[139] While the theories of variance in Schuman resonance are controversial, it will be interesting to monitor whether higher Schumann frequencies correlate with collective elevations in human consciousness, especially love and compassion, following tragic world events or events where large groups powerfully come together to pray or meditate to heal the planet or ourselves.

Gregg Braden, who seems to have spread this hypothesis, paints an elaborate picture of the Earth's magnetic field declining ("We're at the lowest point now in terms of magnetics that we have been in the last 2,000 years"). He predicts the fields will reverse (North Pole becomes South, as happened "maybe 9,000 years ago") and that "We are in the early stages of a magnetic reversal." He added— this was around 2010 or '12—that the Schumann resonances (the earth's heart beat) are rising and "we are linked to those fields, our emotions, our speech patterns . . . as well as to the weather patterns." His view is that "time is speeding up . . . Every cell in our body is in resonance, trying to keep time with the heartbeat of . . . our mother earth . . . trying to match that increase, and we perceive that as time speeding up. . . we've got very low magnetics and the pulse of the planet is twice what it was in the mid-1980s."[140]

On the other hand, Dr. Annette Deyhle, Research Coordinator for the HeartMath Institute, stated categorically, in 2017: "There are and always have been 8 different Schumann resonance frequencies. They are the same as they were when first measured in the 1960s."[141]

To summarize, perhaps forces from the Earth's atmosphere as well as intense collective emotions of others can, either one, influence how we feel and behave. The challenge is to trend both in a favorable direction, avoiding a cyclical downfall. If we can shift our thoughts to more compassion and love, and minimize climate change, then perhaps we can stay on this planet longer.

Do you feel our *dormant* DNA is being activated as we make positive conscious and unconscious efforts towards the planet and its inhabitants, or by positive changes in the Earth's resonate field?

KIMBA: Yes, I feel that the frequencies flooding on the planet now are activating dormant codings in our DNA and are increasing the rate of consciousness evolution, for sure. It is like stimulating a birthing process on the level of consciousness. That is why sound can be helpful . . . it can be the midwifing tool to help make the process smoother and more harmonious. Birth happens, midwife or not . . . but with the right tools the process can be joyful, even ecstatic.

FRED: Agree. I find it refreshing to see the new studies that refute the Darwinian theory that it can take generations to produce adaptation. This supports your belief, and mine, that DNA changes can occur within our lifetime, or in a generation, and not only over thousands of years as more traditionally taught.

An example being that of the *Geospiza fortis* birds on the Galápos Islands—180 of 1,200 of whom lived through a drought by adapting their beaks. And that evolutionary change was passed to the next generation. Now we know that a finch can modify its beak on the fly *during its lifetime* to adjust to availability of seeds and survive. It wasn't necessarily the physically strongest that survived; rather that stronger species can bring about adaptation in real time in a rapid manner. I'm sure that we too can favorably activate our DNA if we pay attention to epigenetic and nutrigenomic modifiers within our control. In other words, if we can maintain a healthier lifestyle and nutrition, we can enhance our DNA health and our longevity. This holds true for sound too. Noise pollution will raise your stress-related cortisol levels, accelerating aging, whereas calming or stimulating music will lower cortisol levels and stimulate new neural synapses.

Thank you for your time and thoughts, Kimba, and I look forward to seeing you perform again soon!

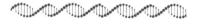

Over many lunches at Jonathan Goldman's favorite Vietnamese restaurant in Boulder, he impressed on me the multiple benefits of simply humming, as laid out in his 2017 book, *The Humming Effect, Sound Healing for Health and Happiness*, coauthored with Andi Goldman. No exotic instruments are needed—just your voice. Physiological benefits are numerous:

- Increased lymphatic circulation

- Lowered blood pressure and heart rate

- Increased melatonin, the hormone that helps you drop into deep sleep

- Reduced levels of the stress-hormone cortisol (high levels can make your brain shrink and make you gain weight)

- Increased endorphins, the hormones that improve mood, pleasure, and are natural pain relievers

- Increased levels of nitric oxide (NO), which dilates blood vessels and lowers blood pressure

- Increased levels of oxytocin, the "trust and love hormone"

A 2011 study from the National Institute of Mental Health and Neuroscience in India found a reduction in stress and blood pressure from Om chanting.[142] Don Campbell, author of *The Mozart Effect: Tapping the Power of Music to Heal the Body, Strengthen the Mind, and Unlock the Creative Spirit*, states that "Humming actually massages the body from the inside out."[143]

In summary, sound can be a healer and, in my opinion, a DNA modifier/shapeshifter. Modalities to resonate frequencies and music include modern high-tech and traditional, often ancient, means—both equally effective. Reducing stress and inflammation through resonate sound with positive intentions can turn off, or dampen, the harmful genes and activate healing genes. The frequency that opens your heart may not be the same as the one needed by your neighbor, but being willing to explore to find your unique resonance will take you to a new level of healing. Sound therapy should be a part of our everyday life, whether simply listening to music on the way to work or having a healer circularly breathing the resonance of a didjeridu on your root chakra. Finding the alchemy of sound, light, and other therapies mentioned in this book will help transform you to a new, healthier being. Expand your playlist and explore this infinite world that awaits you.

Chapter 6

Flowing Your Genome with Water to Optimize Your Health

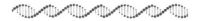

*The ocean stirs the heart, inspires the imagination
and brings eternal joy to the soul.*

—Robert Wyland, Ocean and Whaling Wall artist

Water has always fascinated me—beginning with its molecular structure and ability to form unique crystalline snowflakes, extending to its role in the genesis of life, all the way down to shaping the double helix of our DNA. (I'll detail its intimate role with DNA and the genesis of life later in this chapter.) As humans, we feel this intimate relationship within us and around us. We are drawn to water for survival and spiritual enhancement. Japanese researcher Masaru Emoto, the author of *The Secret Life of Water*, poetically describes this relationship: "You are the water and the wisdom of water, you know. So just allow yourself to flow and then the wonder grows

. . . your soul will reach beyond the seas, with harmony on prayers of peace, never stopping, never halting, bravely water flows . . . Brightly and boldly into the cosmos, for water knows."[144]

Wallace J. Nichols, author of *Blue Mind: The Surprising Science That Shows How Being Near, In, On, or Underwater Can Make You Happier, Healthier, More Connected, and Better at What you Do*, concurs, writing, "It can also help us access the state of 'flow' allowing us to access the default-mode network/daydreaming of our brains while restoring our ability to focus and perform cognitive and creative tasks with greater ease."[145]

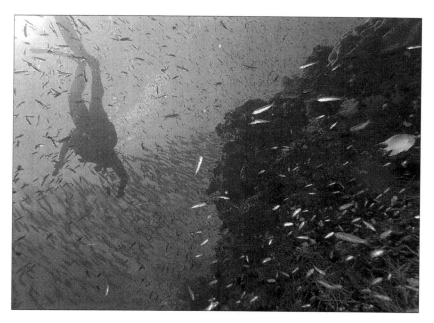

Diving at Fiji. Photo by the author

In 1987, I was nearing college graduation at a small liberal arts school in north Texas. I'd maintained some level of sanity by strategically focusing my pre-med undergrad studies in field biology, rather than being stuck in a lab, doing comparative anatomy. This gave me opportunities to be in nature, instead of being restricted to a lab, predominately fluorescent-lit, staring through a microscope. During an elective in Costa Rica my professors took us out to howl at coyotes and hike amongst exotic birds and monkeys. Escaping to the Pacific coast one summer, I took an underwater marine biology course at the University of California San Diego. Here I studied and photographed the mating habits of the garibaldi fish by diving the golden kelp "forests" just a few hundred yards offshore from La Jolla. Despite this diversity, I desperately desired a more frequent reconnection with the ocean to nourish my soul.

For a few years during childhood, I'd lived near the beach in southern California and, whenever possible, made an annual trip to scuba dive and windsurf in the Pacific, Gulf of Mexico, or Caribbean—not to mention windsurfing on the Gulf Coast during summer break. But this sporadic exposure was not enough to satisfy my sense of a primordial connection with the ocean. Rather than simply lounging on the beach, I have always felt a need to swim, immerse myself with a tank on my back, or feel the waves with a board underfoot.

After college, I was fortunate to live in Hawaii for a year.

Within a few weeks of receiving my BS in biology, I had booked my flight to Oahu and arrived at my aunt's, just a quarter mile from Kohala beach.

My cousin Mike, an excellent surfer, quickly got me up to speed. I was excited to both windsurf and surf Hawaii with him and his buddies.

Late one afternoon in August, I was alone on Diamond Head except for a few locals. I'd been enjoying incredible rides, surfing the fair-sized waves. I've always felt an amazing rush and connection to the ocean, riding waves, being immersed in the embryonic salt water. The kinetic energy flashing across my body amplifies as I paddle out to the break. Catching a wave and feeling the accelerating force underfoot provides yet another sensation, which drives the intimacy of nature deeper into me. Similar to the feeling of a barefoot walking meditation, but there is a more powerful linkup occurring as the kinetic energy of a wave accelerates it into towering height and speed, and it's often borne hundreds of miles away by winds. When I find this optimal wave energy, I'm launched out of my comfort zone, disconnecting my mind chatter and letting me be one with the element. It's common among lovers of outdoor sports—kayaking, windsurfing, kiteboarding, skiing, rock climbing, etc.—to feel this way: "in the zone," or flow. It can be a blissful adrenaline rush, but when we lose focus on our dance with nature, it can mean a fall or wipeout!

After a few hours out I was tired but content, somewhat similar to how you feel after great sex. Catching my last wave, I paddled in, my arms and shoulders heavy. Approaching the lava rocks, as I came off my board I felt something unusual. Luckily, it wasn't a sea urchin or stingray barb in my foot. I was walking knee deep in the current, and the water embraced me. Almost as if confronted by a supernatural force, I was suddenly *stopped*. Instead of resisting the inertia, I yielded to a sensation of acceptance and timelessness. This expanded into a deeper oneness with the ocean and Mother Earth. To the west, the sun was setting, and when I turned east I saw the full moon just emerging over the cobalt-blue ocean. At this magical moment the globe of the full moon and sun were, in tandem, *rising and setting on opposite horizons.* Funny, I thought I was simply going to walk up onto the beach and to my car, but instead I was in a state of spiritual bliss.

But what caused such an impact? As I have reflected back on this moment, I feel confident that through the water the Earth itself was resonating into my body—energetically resonating my DNA to my primal roots. Not only to our planet, but to the delicate harmony of life sustained by the sun, moon, and universe surrounding us. Callum Roberts in his book *The Ocean of Life* expresses this primal connection. He writes: "Our relationship with the sea stretches back through time much further than this: all the way to the origins of life itself. We are creatures of the ocean." Jacques-Yves Cousteau, world-famous oceanographer, adds, "The sea, once it casts its spell, holds one in its net of wonder forever." And, "People protect what they love."[146]

Cousteau goes further, saying, "From birth, man carries the weight of gravity on his shoulders. He is bolted to earth. But man has only to sink beneath the surface and he is free."[147] The field of the water had captured me that evening, and I am forever thankful for that timeless moment.

In the mid-'90s my wife and I were diving on the remote island of Sipadan, offshore from Borneo in the South Pacific. There for a week, we enjoyed four dives daily in the company of fellow divers from around the world. Each dive brought a unique encounter with sea turtles, sharks, frog fish, and many more.

One morning it was with the largest school of barracuda I'd ever seen. Easily two hundred—schooling underwater in a perfect vortex, creating a cone of silver—with the opening *a full fifty feet above me* near the surface. Feeling sure the only chance of a bite would come if I had a flashing object on my body, or a string of fish hanging off my weight belt, I made an intuitive decision to approach the lower end of the vortex *in about sixty feet of water*. Seemed like a crazy thing to do, considering how deep it was, but I didn't feel afraid. As I entered the vortex, the fish didn't scatter, but continued to school around me in the same spinning pattern. A oneness with nature flowed through my body. From thirty feet away, my wife nervously observed me disappear into the encircling school. Luckily, she could see my bubbles flowing to the surface as I spent several minutes relishing in the rotating movement of nature. The wall of silver fish with crooked, sharklike teeth remained undisturbed by my alienlike diver presence. Would they have dispersed had I entered in a state of fear or an intention to hunt them? I'll never know. Observing patterns of schooling fish is similar to watching flocks of starlings fly. They connect to each other and the environment, dancing in unison—with a communal intelligence we seem to have forgotten. Observing and feeling their flow so intimately is a primal experience.

More recently, I was shore diving off the southwest region of Maui, not far from Molokini Island. With my heavy tank, fins in hand, I walked across the lava rocks and cautiously entered through a sandy section into a beautiful cove. My wife was right behind me; being chest deep, we felt relieved of our heavy tanks as we became weightless aquanauts, lightly inflating our buoyancy compensators as we descended and leveled out above the reef, which was teeming with fish. Descending to a shallow depth—of thirty feet or so—we watched the playful sea turtles, along with the Moorish idol fish, triggerfish, and other creatures swimming amongst the lava flows and rose coral. When I descended another thirty feet down and was about halfway through my tank, I heard a symphony of humpback whales transmitting through the waters as if they were right next to me. Based on the intensity, I imagined they were a hundred yards or less away. I'd heard them before on many dives and snorkeling and swum close to them while windsurfing, but this was unique.

The eerie sound of the singing pod flowed through me, connecting me to them as if I were swimming with them. I could hear a shorter, higher-pitched sound—likely was a newborn calf. My wife and I confirmed that we felt a oneness with the ocean and its inhabitants after that dive. Could the resonate tones have touched our deeper energy bodies in ways we couldn't explain? Amongst all whales, the humpback song seems to relate more harmoniously to humans, perhaps even sending messages beyond our conscious perceptions.

According to the British Columbia research project, The North Coast Cetacean Society (NCCS), over a period of more than forty years

> [their] researchers have been following a complex underwater [whale] song that is constantly shifting and reshaping as each season passes. This song, which can range anywhere from 10–30 minutes long, is performed solely by male humpback whales—but for a reason that currently eludes scientists. During the song, humpbacks produce an in-

tricate series of sounds ranging from high-frequency squeals to deep, low-frequency rumbles. The structure is rigid and predictable, and researchers have deconstructed its components into hierarchal elements. The base units (or notes) are singular units of sound, which are linked together to form what is referred to as a sub-phrase. Sub-phrases contain 4–6 notes, and a pair of these groupings is called a phase. Humpbacks tend to repeat phrases perfectly over and over for up to 4 minutes, and the repetition of a select [sic] phrases leads to a theme. The male humpback song is then composed of a collection of various themes, repeated in specific order, delivered with similar musical devices, which are similar to that of a human song, for example, where the emphasis is on the variation in tempo, and the crescendo. As far as we know, humpback whales are the only animals, other than humans, to create such complex, hierarchal patterns of sound.

What makes the song even more fascinating is its evolution between seasons. In any given area, in any given period of time, all singers will perform nearly identical versions of the song. It is most commonly sung during the mating season, but undergoes surprising transformations between years. Sometimes the song will only change subtly, which is revealed by a slight variation in tone or volume. In consecutive other years, the song is almost unrecognizable. Sections may completely disappear, and new themes become incorporated. Regardless of the scale of change, however, all singers within the same geographical region will adopt the same adjustments.[148]

In *Animal Spirits*, anthropological archaeologist Professor Nicholas Saunders (University of Bristol) comments further on the complexity of the song: "The rhythms and refrains of the humpback whale, with a million information-carrying changes of frequency, represent the single most elaborate vocal display in the natural world."[149] What is also amazing is how in the fall the Alaskan cetaceans navigate 3,000 miles to Hawaii for winter, mate, deliver their calves, experience aloha, and return 3,000 miles to the cold, krill-rich waters of the North Pacific.

So what's so spiritual about a whale song? I feel it creates deeper connectedness amongst the pod, perhaps giving them a collective consciousness that guides them the long distances for migration. As they tap into the electromagnetic signatures of Earth, perhaps they add additional acoustic information for the calves. This creates DNA expression in their cortex and energy body, facilitating learning the route. Whale retinas contain biomagnetite, which helps them see the electromagnetic lines on the ocean floor. I feel the combination of sight, sound, and other electromagnetic sensors provides the ultimate GPS.

Like humans, whales also possess pineal glands, but the pineal has been hypothesized by scientists to have a role only in the circadian rhythm and mating season. Perhaps its role is much deeper than currently known, relating to expanded consciousness and intuition.

From a human perspective, when we hear the sound of a whale underwater, particularly a humpback, it automatically resonates. Could we have—passed down to us over thousands of years—an inherited recognition of the tones, or is there more to the resonance subconsciously?

In the spring of the late '80s, I made an adventurous road trip with a good friend, Eric, to Cabo San Lucas (Cabo). This wasn't an easy undertaking, but a 3,500-mile round trip with over seventy hours of narrow, windy roads. We embarked from Durango, Colorado, in my Volkswagen Jetta, loaded up with camping and windsurf gear and a box of our favorite music cassettes. The objective was to enjoy the desert landscape en route, camp in the wilderness, and windsurf and dive the unique ecosystems of the Baja California Peninsula. After a week of poorly paved, narrow, rugged roads, campsite rattlesnakes, fish tacos, Corona beers, REM tunes, and beautiful stops, we reached the tip, with the El Arco (Land's End) rock formation visible from the shores. From Cabo we drove to the beach on the Pacific side and unloaded my gear. Rigging up my sail, I felt a bit nervous about entering the cool waters where the Pacific and Sea of Cortez meet. With its strong currents and a heavy surf entry, there's danger aplenty. Many swimmers have drowned near the point, just a hundred yards away—overwhelmed by the currents. The wind was perfect, though. I couldn't resist.

I made the entry into knee-deep water with my right hand holding the foot straps of my board and my left guiding the sail and boom gracefully. As the wind began to pick up, it lifted me bodily out of the water, allowing me to stand and slide into the foot straps, then begin to glide at a good 20 knots. I maneuvered between a couple large rocks just fifty feet offshore and found myself in heaven as my small board danced me out a half mile into the open blue. I jibed (a downwind turn) and made several runs back and forth. Flying fish were gliding out in front. The board would accelerate underfoot as I came down the wave's front sides and I'd loosen up my sail to feel the momentum. The wind began accelerating, and I was feeling a bit overpowered because of the large sail I'd selected. Suddenly, a gust caught me from behind, catapulting me forward—off the board, twenty feet in front of it. No time to pop my harness line free from the boom as it sent me flying forward!

Hitting the water with a skimming splash, I quickly sighted my board drifting away. Making an intense sprinting swim, I reached my board, which is also my life raft. The waves became larger, wind gusted stronger, and I was struggling to get back on and sail to shore a couple hundred yards away. Holding my board tight, saving up my energy, I patiently waited for a more consistent wind to attempt another start. Five minutes passed, and I was getting nervous as the current began to pull me south. Out of nowhere two large shadows darted under me. I assumed the worst. Great whites, looking for tasty gringo dinner. To limit my limb exposure, I hastily scrambled onto my small board and prepared for impact. Instead, to my delight, a couple dolphins emerged on either side of me from the deep. It was a beautiful sight to see misty spray coming from their blowholes, rather than gaping shark teeth. Seemed like angels from heaven had sent them to help. I couldn't believe they showed, since typically I would have seen them playing around in the open ocean. They stayed another five minutes, comforting me, and soon I was able to come up on my board and sail in safely to the peninsula beach, with them following behind. Walking back towards Eric, I realized something beyond explanation had again occurred.

Dolphins have been known to help humans struggling in the high seas in numerous historical accounts from the Greeks to modern time. One recent case in the Red Sea documented the survival of twelve scuba divers, who floated thirteen hours in the open ocean, awaiting rescue. They were surrounded by a pod of dolphins that repelled several sharks, then jumped in the air as the rescue vessel approached. Dolphins have also helped beached whales return to sea. Scientists hypothesize that the protectionism towards humans may be due to their recognition of a similar skeletal structure through sonar visualization. I feel it is more complex and may be recognition all the way down to the energy field of our DNA. Texas A&M scientist Dr. David Busbee has noted that the human and dolphin genome are basically the same. "It's just that there are a few chromosomal rearrangements that have changed the way the genetic material is put together."[150]

Was I simply just another lucky swimmer, or had they intelligently sensed my distress beyond a sonar evaluation of my physical body? Since I wasn't yelling underwater, perhaps they felt the energetic stress signal from my body, and given humankind's similar DNA and vibrational fingerprint, they were instinctively signaled to rescue me.

What is it in water that resonates and helps connect us to nature and other planetary species? Is it simply that we are bodies made up of 69 percent water or is it the alchemy of water and DNA that links us together?

Water supports us internally both physiologically and spiritually. Physiologic support includes thousands of processes, but on a basic level allows us to reproduce; ensures cellular health and energy; assists in hormone and neurotransmitter production, oxygen delivery, saliva for digestion, bodily waste elimination through urine, temperature regulation; acts as a shock absorber for the brain and spinal cord, and much more. Immersion in it, whether we are soaking in a hot spring or swimming in the ocean, can lower stress hormones like cortisol and relax us. The Director of National Aquatics and Sports Medicine Institute at Washington State University, Bruce Becker, states, "During immersion, the body sends out a signal to alter the balance of catecholamines [adrenal hormones] in a manner that is similar to the balance found during relaxation or meditation."[151] Furthermore, on-going research confirms that stress causes adverse epigenetic changes (modifies your DNA) to your brain and body. So, water as well as many of the other stress-reducing strategies mentioned in this book will support and trend you towards healthier genes.

A 2012 study by Richard Hunter in *Frontiers of Neuroscience* concluded: "It is already clear that stressful interactions with the environment induce regionally and developmentally specific changes in behavior and in brain structure and function. It is also apparent that many of these changes are potentially reversible via environmental or pharmacologic interventions."[152]

Going deeper, a 2011 German study showed that "water molecules surround DNA in a very specific way." This sheath-like relationship helps DNA form the double helix spiral structure and can make it fold and change shape beneficially. That can affect its ability to express proteins, bind drugs, and more.[153]

On a global scale, water synergistically bonds to our DNA, allowing it to morph into the building blocks for amino acids and beyond. Without it, our chromosomes would never have formed, and life would not exist on our planet. Interestingly, water spirals up our strands of DNA, in a way similar to how yogis as early as in the Vedic Upanishads describe the pattern of kundalini energy—on a much larger scale—ascending our spine. Could DNA be awakened similarly to kundalini? Perhaps kundalini awakening resonates and ripples this pattern into our DNA.

The *geometry* of water is also important. Its quality can be influenced by whether water cascaded down a mountain stream or flowed through a city-water recycling system and was pumped through miles of pipes. Beginning in 1994, Dr. Emoto froze samples at minus-25 degrees centigrade in petri dishes. They were observed under a microscope at two hundred times magnification at minus-5 degrees centigrade. He found snowflake-like geometry was much more beautiful, complex, and symmetrical in samples coming from mountain streams.[154]

Jonathan Goldman, in his book *The 7 Secrets of Sound Healing*, rev. ed., gives in-depth insight about this topic, citing in particular the change in the polluted water at the Fujiwara Dam (Japan). At first it photographed looking like mud. But then a priest chanted and prayed over it for an hour. The result? See below the dramatic beauty that emerged.[155]

Even city water, Emoto noted, if being prayed to or spoken to with love, compassion, gratitude, could be transformed to more beautiful geometric forms.[156] Has city water adversely affected both our physical and our spiritual well-being? Can we enhance the water we drink or bathe in? We now see that the Greeks, Romans, Turks, and others really were onto something, in creating healing baths from hot mineral springs. Not only do hot springs have mineral benefits, but also, the geometry is likely enhanced as it flows up from the igneous hot spots below. For those of us not fortunate enough to reside by a mountain stream or hot spring, we can take other measures to improve the quality and energy properties of our water supply.

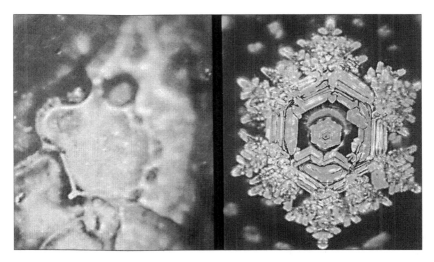

Left Side: Polluted water from Fujiwara Dam.
Right Side: Geometric impact of Buddhist monk chanting
"Heart Sutra" to the polluted water.
Photos by Masaru Emoto from *Messages from Water.*

Some animals have it better than others too. Canoeing on Lewis Lake in Yellowstone on a crisp fall morning several years ago, I had an interesting encounter. My daughter at the bow, son in the middle, and me navigating, we meandered around this scenic lake all by ourselves. We had paddled near the natural outflow of the lake and noticed a hot spring pool in the distance. As we paddled in closer, we witnessed a few elk having a spa day! Half immersed in the steamy water, they were relaxing and content as we floated by. Had hoped to see an elk massage-therapy area adjacent, but wasn't lucky enough to witness that! Animals, including elk, primates, and others, know the benefits of thermal healing water too!

Even if our city water has been classified as "clean and safe" for consumption, does that also hold true for the energetic properties of the water and its ability to resonate with our bodies? As we drink it, will it align with our regenerating cells, forming a healthy hydration shell with our DNA? How do the additives of fluoride, chlorine, and contaminates of other chemicals, plastics, prescription medications, pesticides affect the ability of water to form a healthy bond to our DNA? Could tainted water be more concerning than currently believed?

On the one hand, have humans evolved rapidly enough in the past century to eliminate these new toxins through kidney and liver metabolism? Or on the other hand, are we accumulating this waste in our genome? Dieter Kunz (in Germany) and Jennifer Luke (in England) have in separate research proposed that excessive fluoride in water may lead to calcification of our pineal gland, resulting in hormonal imbalances and declines in melatonin production.[157]

My recommendation is that we do all we can to promote clean water in our local and global communities and drink water that has undergone additional filtration to clear residual chemicals. Support the nonprofit organizations that look out for illegal dumping of chemicals in streams. And work with legislators on clean-water proposals. Unfortunately, our government is insufficiently monitoring your water. This was tragically noted in the lead poisoning of citizens of Flint, Michigan, due to incompetent local and federal management.

Pay close attention to the water we are swimming and bathing in. (Aside: FDR got paralyzed by swimming in a water contaminated with polio virus.) The skin is the largest organ in the body and with its extensive surface area can sponge up toxins. It is difficult to assess the tipping point that may manifest itself as inflammation, cancer, or other disease. People have different genetic capabilities to detox.

How can we promote healthy DNA and gain spiritual benefit from water? Simply start by consuming clean water. If you have access to clean spring or well water in a rural area, then you are in luck! If you live in a large city like me, consider a quality filter or purchase purified spring water in a glass container. Sounds out there, but I have a small tea ball filled with crystals that I place in the base of my glass pitcher to help restructure water as well. Consider a filter for the whole house or at your showerhead to protect yourself further.

Connect to the energy of healthy bodies of water. Visit a nearby park and meditate or hike by a stream or waterfall. Take a swim in a pristine lake or ocean. If the ocean is suffering from a recent oil spill, red tide, brown tide, or other contaminate, then please swim elsewhere, and support local preventative and clean-up efforts. If you see numerous dead fish on a river or sandy beach, frequent tar-balls, or other concerning debris, think twice about swimming in that location. If you are a fisherman like me, don't eat fish from potentially contaminated streams.

Swim safely and connect to the sound, flow, and feel of the water. As environmentalist and author John Muir ("Father of the National Parks System"), who early advocated to preserve our wildernesses, advised, "Take a course in good water and air; and in the eternal youth of Nature you may renew your own."[158]

The vibrational frequency of flowing water is healing and emits negative ions that are calming to our energy fields. "All life flows with the flow of water," Emoto reminded us.[159] *While meditating on the shore, visualize the water cleansing your body and resonating your DNA to optimal health.* Breathe in the fresh air and vaporized water to cleanse your lungs and open your heart. Be one with the molecule you are mostly made of and nurture its purity and energetic qualities for your health.

Chapter 7

The Power of Dancing Your DNA!

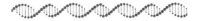

Let's dance
Put on your red shoes and dance the blues
Let's dance
To the song they're playin' on the radio
Let's sway
While color lights up your face
Let's sway
Sway through the crowd to an empty space

—**David Bowie**, "Let's Dance"

Expression through dance has been natural to humans and many animals since creation. What is its purpose? It's sometimes part of a courting ritual, as illustrated in the colorful mating dance of Birds-of-Paradise; or it can serve to achieve an ecstatic state, as with the whirling of a dancing dervish, or to please a particular god or goddess.

Most of us simply enjoy being in synch with music and one another! As we observe young children moving to sound, with rhythm or beat, dance seems instinctual. We are likely to be more graceful in our prime years, then less fluid as we age. Without a doubt, my patients who keep dancing well into their eighties are in the best of health. In addition to physical benefits, there are deep spiritual and energetic elements, which I believe help us express a healthier genome and promote longevity.

Dance's primal roots go back thousands of years. Native Americans danced to summon rain and to help insure adequate food, reproduction, and survival, when faced with threats from the environment and war.

The Sun Dance is still practiced by Native Americans of the Great Plains. This dance requires stamina, often including piercing the skin on the chest of men, who, despite being tethered to a cottonwood "tree pole" (sun pole), dance ceremonially to the hypnotic drumbeat of the tribe.[160] The sun pole was selected, felled, and installed in the center of the circle, with a thunderbird nest placed on top. As anthropologist George A. Dorsey described this event celebrated by the Ponca Nation of Oklahoma in 1902, with yellow-painted bodies, crowned with crow or hawk feathers, grasping sage in their right hand, and attached by the chest with rawhide thongs to the pole, they danced for days.[161] Buffalo, eagle, and crow are represented, alongside offerings of tobacco in the ceremonial pipe. The various songs and dances—passed down by generations—push the dancers to their physical limits, while connecting them to Spirit.

The event typically lasts four to eight days. Overall, the purpose is to show respect to Mother Earth and the cycles of life, death, regeneration. Participants believe that spiritual rebirth of the tribe and Earth may occur or at least be promoted through this ceremony. During the fasting, drumming, and prolonged dancing, visions often arise. Deeper elements of this ceremony are kept secret, not shared with the public. Once outlawed by the U.S. and Canadian governments, the Sun Dance is protected by the American Religious Freedom Act of 1978.[162] We can only hope that—except in the eventuality of significant threat to life—this tradition, and the dances and ceremonies of thousands of other indigenous cultures, will continue for centuries without hindrance.

I love to dance, but I have to admit, after blowing out my Achilles doing a 360-degree dance move in 2016, I was humbled and decided I should interview those with a deeper knowledge of graceful dance, so that I might enhance my own moves, help others, and return to the dance floor . . . baby.

I've always been intrigued by the natural flow of qigong and Tai Chi of Asia, as well as the Polynesian hula. As much as I'd love to write about them all, it would take another book to do so!

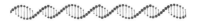

The Art, Energy, and Wisdom of Qigong
(A Chinese meditative movement/dance)

Based on such evidence as depictions on a Neolithic vessel, the gymnastic and shamanic meditative roots of qigong likely go back 7,000 years.[163] To learn more about this powerful tradition, I questioned an expert, Jef Crab, founder of the international E.AS.T. (Energetic Awareness, Sensitivity and Transformation)

Institute. A Belgian national, in 1984, he set out from Europe to Taiwan in search of the source of movement.

> [There] he was accepted by Master Wang Hui Jun (Henry), who was already at that time multiple Pushing Hands champion of the Taiwan Tai Chi Association. From this encounter he abandoned all outer-style martial arts and dedicated himself to study solely inner movement . . .
>
> In those years he also had a very close contact with the world-famous Sumi-e and Ikebana teacher Akira Tatsumura, a Zen Master who mentored him on the deeper aspects of the mind and the energetic layers. Several times Jef stayed for longer periods in the Tatsumura residence in Milan and was instructed privately.
>
> His journey to the source of all movement finally brought him to the Hungarian shaman Jóska Soós de Sóvar, himself born into the Basci clan, the Hungarian shaman clan with roots to Siberian Shamanism. This first meeting was the result of dreams in which Jóska, at the time unknown to Jef, appeared so dramatically and with such accuracy that, two years later, Jef found his way to Jóska's home in Antwerp.[164]

FRED: What do you think, Jef? How old are the roots of qigong?

JEF: They date from a few million years ago. In my opinion the slow movements of taiji were derived from stalking game. While stalking, the hunter has to maintain an enormous body awareness, keeping his balance, controlling every movement (even the slightest). He has to sense the environment and, of course, the inner state of the game itself: *is it still unaware of his presence or is already beginning to sense a sort of, yet undefined, danger?* Of course, our understanding of these movements was never so sophisticated as in our present days. The contemporary taiji masters have a much clearer perception than our predecessors did on the origin of the movement. No doubt about that. Their understanding of, e.g., muscle cycle and the ability to store energy and release it again—the so-called *fa jin technique*—has much refined over the centuries.

We can still observe today that taiji, and qigong are natural movements. Especially when we observe predators like lions, big cats, lizards, or spiders, etc. They have the ability to move slowly toward their prey and then suddenly explode. A cheetah reaches a speed of sixty-five miles an hour in less than three seconds. Also, in other martial arts many of the famous masters through the ages claim that their movements already existed in nature.

"The movements in Ai Ki Do are the movements of nature which form a deep and infinite mystery. Those who understand yet anything of this secret understand deeply that man himself is the image of the Universe"—O-Sensei Ueshiba Morihei.

It couldn't be different, as we directly originate from nature. All our abilities, energy, and life processes are derived directly from nature. It is common knowledge that this is the case for breathing and digesting, but also our nervous system was first developed in the plant world and later refined in the animal kingdom.

FRED: I've heard that in the West, in particular the U.S., "qigong still carries the magic and the mystery from the Old World, unlike yoga, which has been more commercialized. And because of that, qigong is still rife with a deep spiritual wisdom it's bringing to us."[165] What wisdom would this be, condensing down to a crucial point?

JEF: We have to assume that the knowledge people gained from their lives, as far back as the first humanoids millions of years ago, is what we today call shamanic. They never called it that. It was simply their knowledge to live in a certain environment. Six million years, they were walking together with big predators like raptors, sabretooths, cave bears, and other threats on the savannahs. From a point of view of physical strength they had very little or no chance to survive normally. They had to find other abilities. They had no time for philosophy. They only had time to live together.

Consequently, we had to think in terms of a group, like antelopes or buffalo. Thus, our ancestors unintentionally created a group energy. This made us win over the predators constantly preying on us and hunting us. From being able to connect to this group energy and experiencing its power, shamanic techniques developed. It is in the understanding of connecting to *successive deeper or larger layers of consciousness and energy* they developed what master shaman Joska Soos called the five axes, one of the fundamentals of shamanism. Also, in contemporary taiji and qigong we know that connecting to the larger sphere creates power.

FRED: How are Taoism—and any of your other practices (taiji, qigong, shamanism)—connected to health in a way that's missing from the Western approach?

JEF: Well, only nature heals. And life itself decides which forms—expressions of life—will continue to evolve and which have to dissolve (I don't use the word *die*, because we transform into something else). So Tao is the way of nature; it's this movement that carries us through a lifetime of growth. But at a certain moment we have to release our life energies and give them back to nature. It's not dying. That's a Christian or Catholic opinion about an interrupted cycle. In shamanism and Taoism we only see the cycle. Dying is only a moment of transformation. So through Taoism we understand that the only thing the healer can do is try to stimulate this inner attitude in the patient, in order that nature can do this work again, to connect to the patient's own healing force instead of connecting to the other side: trauma, etc.

FRED: On a more everyday level, on the Universal Healing Tao Center website of Master Mantak Chia, I find this explanation:

> In the Taoist tradition, positive and negative emotions are associated with the internal organs. One of the keys to good health is to become aware of the emotional energies that reside in the organs, and to transform the negative emotional energies into positive virtues. Taoists believe that we are all born with the virtues of love, gentleness, kindness, respect, honesty, fairness, justice, and righteousness. . . .
>
> In the Tao "emotional intelligence" is a process of recognizing emotions by their effects on the body, and employing exercises that transform the negative emotions into positive life force, or Chi. Two important exercises are the "Inner Smile" and the "Six

Healing Sounds" techniques, as taught by Master Mantak Chia.

What role do spiritual healers or I, as a physician, play in this process?

JEF: One example is where you can bring the patient to such a state of relaxation—take away what is blocking this relaxation and energy flow in the body—that the person can connect to the healing force of nature. It is not important how, by what technique or method, this is achieved. The process can even be supported by herbal or chemical medicine, if necessary.

FRED: Studies by cell biochemist Glen Rein in the 1990s go to that point, about relaxation, Rein wanted to target DNA to test whether healers could affect biology. He began to work with the HeartMath Research Center, demonstrating the effect of emotions on our DNA. In one study, where he partnered with Rollin McCraty, the research director of the Institute of HeartMath, twenty-eight researchers trained in coherent heart emotion emanated anger, love, etc., toward twenty-eight human placenta tissue vials; the study noted that the DNA either *relaxed—unwinding and becoming longer*—or tensed (contracted, tightened up, shortened) according to the emotion directed toward it.

> Even more relevant, when the strands tightened due to the negative feelings, many of the DNA codes previously available switched off. Once the strands were sent positive intentions of gratitude, the effects of the negative feelings were reversed and the "shut down" DNA codes were switched on again.

What's interesting is the fact that positive feelings have a much greater effect on DNA than negative feelings. The reason why has to do with the vibration frequencies of these emotions. Negative emotions such as fear, hate, or anger have lower frequencies, and can be depicted as a loose, wide sine wave that connects to few parts of the DNA strand. Meanwhile positive emotions such as love, happiness, and gratitude have higher frequencies, and can be depicted as a much tighter, narrow sine wave capable of connecting to more parts of the strand.

The research recommends the "science of gratitude."

Five-times *New York Times* best-selling author Gregg Braden commented: "The view that all healing is really self-healing is strongly supported by Glen Rein's inspiring research in DNA's response to coherent emotions."[166]

That's similar to what Masaru Emoto, in *The Secret Life of Water*, described.[167] In that case, water surrounded by someone sending loving thoughts created beautiful snowflake-like geometry, whereas water that met with negative thoughts created less complex, less beautiful geometry.

Elizabeth Wilcock was the first to point out Rein's research to me. She's referred to by many as the "Warrior Priestess of Love," and is the founder and director of the Priestess Path, "a training ground for women who are ready to embody the Divine Feminine and show up as leaders blessing this world." She has owned martial art schools, earned five black belts in Shaolin kung fu, and is the first female master instructor in her organization. Blending in additional East-West expertise in qigong, sexuality, and spirituality makes her a powerful healer to those who resonate with her teachings. We discussed dancing your DNA from a qigong perspective as well as the dance of masculine and feminine energy to make a better, healthier planet.

She connects these studies to the inner *smile* in qigong. Here is how she puts it: "It's scientifically proven. Directed anger, whether I'm angry at myself or I'm angry at you, is going to kill your DNA. The whole teaching of the inner smile in qigong is, *you are going through your entire body and seeing everything as perfect.* You visualize it, and then you're intending it. Dr. Rein demonstrated scientifically that by combining the image of it as perfect and the intention for it to be perfect, there is a 40 percent increase in health. The results even indicated that focused positive human intention can decrease the growth of tumor cells by modulating the DNA synthesis. So intent can change DNA favorably."[168]

Pulling up the 1996 study "Effect of Conscious Intention on Human DNA," I see that Rein concluded:

> This experiment demonstrated that intention produced the same 20% inhibitory effect as did imagery alone. On the other hand, when the image of few cells in the petri dish was combined with the intention for the cells to return to their natural order, the inhibitory effect on cell growth was doubled to 40%.[169]

So, Jef, do you believe that intent can influence qi and also even alter DNA?

JEF: I fully agree with the theory except for one nuance. The *real impression* is made on our energetic being. The shift in DNA is the *result* of changing our energetic being. Meaning that if we became more aware about the energetic and conceptual layer of our being, we could directly transform blocking, inhibiting energies into activating factors without working through the DNA. Also, the fact that DNA does not play the role science assumed is becoming more and more clear. *DNA is not the definer of our being, as it is obviously in constant change, adapting to the environment.* Our energetic state of being is much more important.

FRED: How does one most effectively move qi (life force energy)?

JEF: Life force moves in a natural way. *To let go any kind of block or attachment on the physical, emotional, mental, and spiritual level* would give the best result in having qi moved in and around the body. Hence, the emphasis on remaining relaxed in taiji. Only in this deep, relaxed state can we become aware of the energy flows in and surrounding the body. With correct intention we are more than able to gather and move qi in a certain direction.

ELIZABETH ADDS: In qigong, we believe that optimal health and balance is achieved through the accumulation of light and energy directed by the mind. That's why I like to bring in that particular study from Rein, which shows the science of how the most effective healing tool is our vision of something being perfect and our intention for it to be so. One of the main reasons for doing qigong is to really pull light and energy into our own body. Suck it in from the earth, from the sky, from the sun, from the air; we're literally inhaling, eating the energy. And then storing it in our batteries.

FRED: Through scientific studies and/or your own experiential knowledge, do you feel qigong, taiji, and yoga help us spiritually resonate our DNA into healthy or more energized states?

In his answer, Jef drew in the age-old science of the Tao.

JEF: All movement originates from the Tao—from the Tao it goes through the four lower axes, finally condensing into the physical world. It is not that a human being changes the energetic process. We are only *following the movement*. The thing we can do is to go along with the flow, to *become one with the Tao or block it*. Of course, to me the Taoist movement, taiji, and shamanism are scientific.

FRED: You're referring back to the five axes of shamanism—that developed over millions of years, which therefore must be in our DNA?

JEF: Yes, 1) the physical (connected to the body), 2) the energetic (planet connection), and 3) the conceptual (solar-system connection) are important to our well-being. The fourth is already a healing force (connected further than the solar system). The fifth is what masters call the Tao.

FRED: And the fourth and fifth levels bring in the multidimensional? How would there be a healing force beyond the solar system that relates to human health?

JEF: In shamanism we accept the idea of the Primordial Sound. It is pure energy, pure intention, and pure intelligence. It is pure energy, a vibration. Its vibrations reach throughout the Infinite. Our solar system is just a result of the Primordial Sound. Our origins lay in this sphere. The solar system delivers—as an intermediary—what we call the *conceptual field* for our planet and its inhabitants. Concept meaning *plan*, something that still has to be developed to its full potential.

FRED: And how is your shamanic work connected with sound?

JEF: Sound is vibration. The shamanic healer connects first to the deepest layer or axis according to his ability. Sound works especially from the fourth axis into the third. The shaman travels into the fourth axis level, maybe into the fifth. The master travels into the fifth. But even those who are already able to travel into the third may help others. No doubt about that.

FRED: HeartMath founder Doc Childre has a theory of heart intelligence: that "The heart serves as a key access point through which information originating in the higher dimensional structures is coupled into the physical human system (including DNA) and that states of heart coherence generated through experiencing heartfelt positive emotions increase this coupling." Does this sound right to you?

JEF: Yes it does. With this understanding: that the change is primarily in the energetic complex and that the DNA structure, being mere matter, will follow. "To connect" can only be done on an energetic level. But no doubt, our level of coherence will change our energetic structure.

FRED: Please give me your opinion on how qigong/taiji may favorably enhance DNA or reduce systemic inflammation. A quick note on nomenclature for our readers: Qigong, Qi Gong, Chi Gong, and Chi Kung are the same thing, simply varied spellings. Similarly, Taiji is another spelling for Tai Chi.

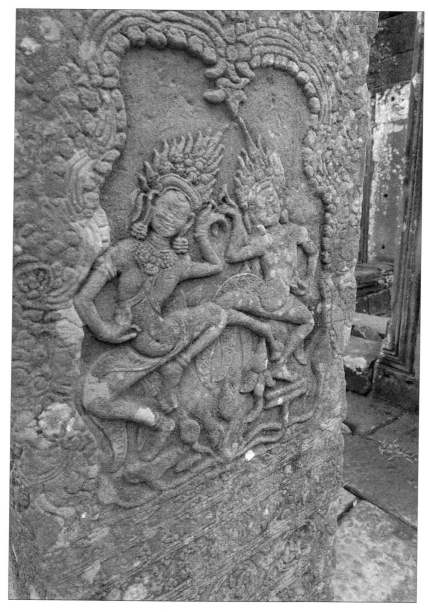

Dancing Apsaras at Angkor Wat. Photo by the author.

JEF: The tradition is clear on the benefits of improving the circulation of qi, vital life force, in the body. Elaborated reports on its workings have been written by various masters. I will not repeat those here.

However, it is my experience that during exercising taiji the mind shifts to deeper levels of consciousness. . . . The deep relaxation that is the result of the exercise alone already has a positive effect on inflammation—under the condition that the practitioner can practice without too much pain. Furthermore, the accompanying state of mind will change the energetic patterns inherited from ancestors and thus change the DNA favorably.

Once again, it is a matter of creating these circumstances in which the healing force of the conceptual layers can penetrate our being again. It is all there already. We just have to accept it.

FRED: To take an example of these "inherited patterns," holocaust-survivor descendants have been found, in tests, to have altered stress hormones.[170] Similarly, a 2017 *Science* article reported that in nematode worms exposed to high temperature the traumatic "ancestral legacy" effects were passed on for up to ten generations.[171] Is that what you mean?

JEF: It is. Just look at a newborn baby. Who teaches it to find its mother's nipple, move its fingers, open its eyes, or cry? All these movements are necessary to develop its energetic structure. Who teaches it to crawl and stand up? We just repeat all the movements from our ancestors. This already begins in the womb at conception. In the womb we will repeat our complete history since the first cell in the primordial ocean up to humanoid. After birth we repeat all the movements our human ancestors already made. All these movements are important.

In Western society we look upon ourselves as individuals, separated from each other, but also separated from the ancestral lineage. This is a misunderstanding. In shamanism we assume that every person carries at least forty generations of his or her ancestors within. All our movements, actions and reactions, thoughts and feelings are more memories and reproductions than "our own" production. And indeed also, their traumatic experiences might influence our decisions.

On the deeper energetic level we literally connect to all living beings . . . even to the solar system. If we manage to follow the Tao, the natural movement, we might contribute something to the evolution of humankind. But only at the end of our life. This is why one of my teachers stated expressly: "There are no young Masters!"

FRED: To that point, a number of fairly recent books talk about qigong as a cancer cure or say that Chinese medicine deals with the whole body, unlike targeted Western medicine. Professor Qian Xueshen, a famous Chinese nuclear physicist, says: *"Research into Qi energy will lead us to the last frontiers of man's understanding of the human body."*[172] Similarly, Michael Winn, President of the National Qigong (Chi Kung) Association of the USA and the founder of Healing Tao University in New York, writes: "While chi kung's medical effectiveness has been well documented in China by scientists for a wide variety of chronic illnesses, the stories of recovery from cancer are among the most frequent and most dramatic. Many patients have been told to go home and die, that not even chemo or radiation (widely used in China today) can help. They go home, and out of final desperation begin doing chi kung movements and meditations. Twenty years later, they are leading classes and writing books on how chi kung saved their life:

Most disease is caused by emotional trauma and lack
of sexual energy flow. This constricts the free flow
of chi in the body. The type of emotion will usually
determine where the tumor will appear. In the weak-
ened areas, tissue begins to form around the stagnant
chi, and then a virus, seeing an area of unconscious-
ness with nobody "living" in that part of the body,
decides to take up residence and grow itself.[173]

The book *Chi Gong: The Ancient Chinese Way to Health*, by Paul
Dong and Aristide H. Esser (1990),[174] is just one that talks about
its beneficial effects on cancer:

One explanation for the sense of serenity produced
by entering a state of deep meditation through chi
gong is the increase in the absorption of oxygen. In
ancient China, Taoist priests chose to meditate under-
neath the pine tree because they had discovered that
the pine exudes the greatest amount of oxygen.[175]

So Chinese medicine treats the whole body. This seems in line
with what you said about relaxation and improving the circulation of qi. Fascinating, isn't it?

Let me ask you one other question, Jef, that relates to carrying old
wounds. In regard to our planet, do you feel the Divine Feminine
is out of balance?

JEF: Not the planet itself. The human species is out of balance.
The dark light of the planet from where all the species on the
planet originate (the energetic womb of all the creatures of this
planet, the creative force, the materia prima) is probably the same

as millions of years ago. But in humans and humanity the relationship of masculine to feminine is not in balance. That's very correct. We can see that in the societal model. *The whole economy is completely out of balance with nature.* Contemporary Western society and it's followers are completely disconnected from nature and therefore from the healing force.

Here, I returned to Elizabeth Wilcock on the subject of connecting in a tribal manner with sound. I wanted her input regarding brain states.

FRED: Elizabeth, how do you feel using a drum and rattle dancing around a fire or in circle differs from doing qigong or yoga in a studio?

ELIZABETH: Well, we know that rhythmic rattling, drumming, rhythmic dancing, rhythmic singing, shifts us into a low alpha, high theta brainwave state, which corresponds to the parasympathetic nervous system. This is also called the shamanic state of consciousness where we can access visionary and deep healing states. When we are dancing and playing or listening to music that induces a trance state, we are accessing this primal limbic state, which is very healthy for us to do.

FRED: Yes, it's important to activate those deeper limbic structures of our brain that are more offline and dormant in modern humans. This trance state takes us into sonic entrainment (or entrancement). As a reminder, entrancement is when brainwaves assume a pattern, such as predominately alpha waves, through sound or light; being entranced together can lead to coherence, or a group—perhaps an audience—feeling connected. Adding in the elements of nature, such as dancing around a fire, on a bluff overlooking an ocean, on sacred sites, and even dressed in costumes or masks of native animal species further amplifies the experience.

ELIZABETH: For sure, when we enter into the low alpha, high theta brainwave state, we enter our visionary states and dream states. Deep healing resides there. It's important that we can access that and do access that. All these old ancient cultures have a way of accessing it. The Maasai jump up and down. You know?

FRED: Indeed, I've danced and jumped with them in Tanzania back in 2012. It's crazy how high they can jump in the Adumu dance! I can't come close. Traditionally this leaping dance has had the purpose of initiating the boy into becoming a warrior man.[176]

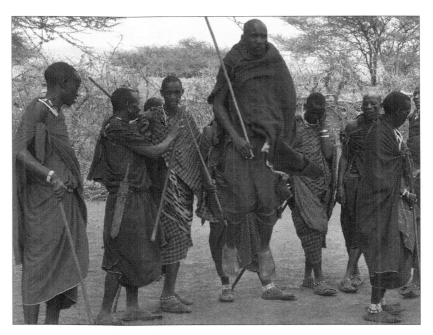

A Maasai doing jumping Adumu Dance, Tanzania. Photo by author

An alternative to jumping is spinning, as seen in the Sufi whirling dervishes that spin themselves into a meditative state to lose their ego, merge with God, or even perhaps to imitate the rotation of planets.

As one writer put it,

> Each dance consists of three stages: the first is the knowledge of God; the second is the seeing of God; and the third is the union with God.
>
> The conical hats the dervishes wear represents a tombstone, the dervish's jacket symbolizes the grave, and the dervish's skirt, a funeral shroud. As the dervishes dance they remove their jackets to show they are shedding earthly ties, and escaping from their graves. As they whirl, the dervishes raise their right hands in prayer and extend their left hands toward the floor. The meaning of these gestures is "what we receive from God, we give to man; we ourselves possess nothing." Their whirling symbolizes the rotation of the universe in the presence of God.[177]

The Sufi spin began with Rumi, the thirteenth-century mystical Persian poet, born in present-day Afghanistan. The story goes that on a walk through a marketplace in Turkey, he became spellbound by the sound of workers hammering gold. Listening to that ritualistic hammering, the story goes, he heard—translating it into English—"There is no god but Allah." In that instant, he was "so entranced in happiness he stretched out both of his arms and started spinning in a circle [Sufi whirling]. With that the practice of *Sama* and the dervishes of the Mevlevi order were born."[178] This entrainment with the hammering is an example of becoming connected to a oneness with the universe. In regard to our planet, do you feel the Divine Feminine is out of balance?

ELIZABETH: Yes, I think one of core problems on Earth is that we're really out of alignment with Divine Feminine energy, all of us. So, look at the Earth, an amazing place. Then you see what we are doing to this Earth. Such as mankind polluting the oceans with toxins.

FRED: Agree, and in addition to the pollution of our air and water, the adverse effects of man-made climate change are devastating our forests and coral reefs. I've witnessed the bleaching of reefs worldwide during my almost forty years of diving. Locally here in Colorado and the mountainous west, pine trees are dying off in the millions as pine and spruce beetles thrive in the milder winters, burrowing into the drought-stricken trees in summer and taking 'em down. I recently read that we've got 834 million standing-dead trees in Colorado since 2010.[179]

ELIZABETH: It's because we haven't really honored her. We've taken advantage of her in so many different ways. The Earth is feminine; the air, water, and soil are all part of the body of the feminine Earth. Animals are also feminine, the Earth's children. What have we done to the whole way of life? The masculine energy, this penetrating energy, has forced an idea on it; it said, *Oh I'm going to take all this fossil fuel out and I'm going to create a fuel source that creates pollution.* Therefore, we have cities you can't even breathe in.

FRED: Acid rain, air and water pollution, rising ocean levels from glacial melt, to mention a few. Folks in Mexico City, Beijing, and New Delhi are dying from respiratory and cardiovascular disease at high rates. Not to mention the extreme weather on the spectrum of drought or flooding, acid rain, air and water pollution, rising ocean levels from glacial melt, to mention a few.

ELIZABETH: We have polluted the feminine, and that is the meta-relationship we have right now with Her. What can we do? Each person has both the yin *and* the yang within them. You're a man; I'm a woman. There's slightly different things we can do to honor the feminine. . . . I really feel the world is thirsting for compassion, sweetness, and understanding. I feel the best thing a woman can do is to try to embody those noble aspects of the feminine, and then with her yang, masculine, protective side, she can stand for the feminine. The masculine, yang counterpart of the feminine stands in protection of her so that she can unfurl in her beauty freely and unviolated. The problem is that we, humanity, are violating the feminine as a whole. We are taking Her resources, we are polluting Her air and Her waters and we are harming the innocents and the animals. The warriors are supposed to stand up and protect the feminine from being violated and misused. Men have typically been those warriors holding a protective space for the women and children to live and play unadulterated. Making a stand in protection of the Feminine is a noble task for any warrior, male or female and we need these warriors now.

FRED: So true. We can only hope that through your work, and the work of other masters cognizant of the world's delicate yin/yang balance that we can shift the planet and its inhabitants to a higher state of compassion and love, thus promoting healing and sustainability. Thank you, Elizabeth, for your time and ongoing work.

Getting back to the original question, Jef, how do you feel using a drum and rattle dancing around a fire or in circle differs from doing qigong or yoga in a studio?

In his answer, Jef emphasizes the importance of a relaxed, embodied energy flow and awareness, by no matter what means.

JEF: The medium or technique is not important. The energy flow from deep subtle layers to more materialized expressions is. My teachers, Akira Sensei and Jóska Soós, expressed healing force through their paintings or in the case of Akira through ikebana, the Japanese art of flower arranging. I developed the E.A.S.T. method to allow people to express healing force through daily-life activities. The *state of mind* of the artist/healer is most important. *That energetic state will be projected and shared with the observers/ participants, influencing their energetic complex.*

The dance would take the individual into a deeper state of mind. Like war dances of Germanic people, Celtic people. It helps the individual be more coherent, more intelligent, softer even. But the real transformation lies in what's happening on a societal level. Take the Dalai Lama. It's about compassionate action . . .

More broadly, there were no tribal wars as Neanderthals. There were only tribal wars when we became "civilized." There is no proof of mass murder until 7,000 years ago, when there were around twenty-six individuals, all ages, killed in a traumatic way. That is the Lake Turkana incident.[180] Before, we seemingly didn't have this, although anthropologists have found skeletons with wounds, in which the wounded person lived on after the accident. This means they were taken care of. We have a lot of scientific proof that the Neanderthal took care of each other.

We are not Neanderthal. Something changed and we became extreme, too individual, and more detached from one another. But I have to connect to my society. Otherwise, as a shaman I cannot tap into these layers. The real transformation comes from acting. In daily life. True healing comes from compassionate action toward our fellow human being and nature.

FRED: To summarize: we need to dance our masculine and feminine energies in ways that will embody flow and benefit the health of the individual and all living beings on this planet. Ultimately, the goal is to find ways—as we coexist amongst each other—to transform or attenuate these darker energies that may be overly penetrative to the planet and individuals, reshaping and flowing them into a beneficial outcome.

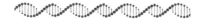

A Unique Perspective from a Former Rave/EDM Dancer

Looking for a modern spiritual perspective on dance that has a great potential to shift our genome—or, as Jef put it, alter our energetic and conceptual layers in ways that "transform blocking, inhibiting energies into activating factors"—I sought out Linda Driscoll Powers, a fifteen-year veteran of the Electronic Dance Music (EDM) scene. EDM represents a large subculture in the U.S. and Europe, and Linda was part of it at its underground inception. The founder of Dance Fitness Fun, Linda is a friend and one of the most passionate, amazing dance instructors in Colorado. She is also a longtime Health & Medical Copywriting & Education contractor and is currently attending the CU College of Nursing with an interest in mental health. Having made the deep dive in this community, she can speak from her heart in regard to this culture.

FRED: Linda, how did you get the fire and passion to make dance such a big part of your daily life?

LINDA: As long as I can remember, I've loved to dance; rhythm has always moved through me in joyful ways. It can't be repressed. I started dancing at three years old—tap and ballet. Even quite young, I thought: *This is it.* As soon as I start dancing, I am overcome with joy. I did really well in formal classes as a child. Practicing was never a chore; I could do it all day long!

As I grew older, I realized that dancing was a powerful therapy. Whenever I felt down or upset, I would dance. I discovered the underground electronic culture—otherwise known as rave culture—in the mid-90s. This environment gave me an outlet to dance for hours on end, until I simply couldn't stand any longer. On rave dance floors, everyone would show up and be their unique selves. It didn't matter what you looked like or what your societal status was, because on the dance floor, we are all equal. We were free from judgment of each other, free from the societal pressures and stress. I really fell in deep and the rave culture became my family.

FRED: I've read that the mostly recreational drug MDMA (3,4-Methylenedioxymethamphetamine) is frequently used in the rave culture. Did you work with it much, and if so what benefits or dangers did you notice?

LINDA: Yes, I experimented with MDMA in the beginning, but grew out of needing exogenous molecules to free my soul on the dance floor. When I first experimented with MDMA and dance, the molecule did help "lift the veil" on my own consciousness. It served like a key in the lock of my spiritual growth in ways that might have taken years and years to uncover otherwise. I, like many people, had early-life traumas—such as the death of my father—that I was struggling to move beyond. I believe that the sparing, responsible use of MDMA, along with vigorous dance in a positive social setting, helped me process the grief and fear, ultimately moving into a space of greater self-love and spiritual security. I am very grateful for that.

FRED: Sounds like you found an alternative solution—deep therapy on the dance floor instead of the traditional office setting of a psychologist.

LINDA: Indeed, it was, and I believe that MDMA has strong potential for use in myriad forms of trauma-recovery therapy, but that's another conversation entirely.

Of course, I had friends who got caught up in the world of intoxicants and were worse off for it. To put it simply: rave culture and electronic social dance is a form of escape from the daily grind. There is no stress on the dance floor—only joy, freedom, and acceptance. That can be a very addicting force, especially when mind-altering substances are thrown into the mix. A few people have died along the way, and that broke my heart.

FRED: So were there heavier drugs being used, such as heroin?

LINDA: Yes, but the heroin isn't connected to MDMA. No way. As in a culture or subculture, there are hurting human beings who seek out ways to blunt their unhealed pain and trauma. One of my friends, an amazing soul and spiritual dancer, became addicted to painkillers after sustaining a head injury in the military. The doctors addressed his physical pain with opioids, but they were unable to address his spiritual needs and PTSD in healthy or effective ways. Talking about his emotional pain was very difficult. He was scared of losing friends because he felt like a monster and was overcome with guilt. Dancing helped a lot, but rave culture is an escape from life—not life itself. He didn't have ways to process his pain during daylight hours. He moved from the VA-prescribed pills to heroin, and it ultimately killed him.

FRED: Right. I'll bet if they had treated his pain without narcotics, using acupuncture and integrative pain-management therapy, he'd most likely be alive today. I read recently that the FDA designated MDMA as "breakthrough therapy" for PTSD in July 2017. This should allow for a faster investigation, building on existing research so that someday soon, veterans and other suffering from PTSD may benefit in a legal and more therapeutically guided way.[181]

LINDA: Yes, no doubt. I stand behind researching these therapies 100 percent.

FRED: It sounds like you experienced an awakening through dance and EDM. Did you feel like you were connecting to God within yourself or God in the upper heavenly-like worlds? How would you describe that?

LINDA: Well, both! I felt like my soul was an energetic force, like a light; one that every other person on this planet has. And that the vibration of our souls makes us equal regardless of human form. We all need love and joy and connection to other humans to thrive. After this awakening, I started to consciously connect with the souls of others with great intention. This practice became a high in and of itself!

FRED: Were you connecting to your higher self, God, Christ consciousness, a state of samadhi or nirvana, or anything that you could identify?

LINDA: Christ consciousness is a good description; I felt connected to a grid of many connected human souls. This grid, or collective consciousness energy, became my sense of God.

FRED: Sounds ecstatic. Do you feel that the gridlike visuals were a form of sacred geometry that was stimulated more by dance, music, or the MDMA?

LINDA: Once the molecule, combined with vigorous dance, opened me up to being able to feel it, I began to practice this state of awareness away from the music and molecules. The practice became an ingrained part of my own consciousness, like a walking meditation. No longer did I need molecules such as MDMA to get me there.

FRED: Good.

LINDA: Later in my life I realized grid patterns were sacred geometry; this then stimulated my interest in Reiki. I achieved Reiki master and continued to seek out new ways to explore my energy body, such as the MerKaBa Meditation.

FRED: That's great that the sacred geometry came through and that you had what sounds like a kundalini awakening. Tell me a bit more about these underground raves.

LINDA: There's a sense of intense connection without saying a word. We *got* each other as we danced with each other, not necessarily touching, but sharing space. It's a whole 'nother world, to walk into a large room where there is well-dialed-in sound that overcomes you to the point where you don't get to have many thoughts of your own, because it's so all-encompassing. You just MOVE and dance and dance and dance. I believe that on the dance floor, our nervous systems and hearts align with a synchronous beat—we become one. It's a beautiful thing!

FRED: Really sounds like you were resonating to group oneness through the dance and sonic(sound) entrancement!

LINDA: Absolutely. And the light. I could see that the light of our souls, and each one of us, made up the larger light of what we call God. I'd been raised in an environment of Christianity and Catholicism that frankly scared me; I thought, *There's no way God could be this vengeful.* I never believed in it and I felt really lost as a result. Since having that first spiritual "aha moment" on the dance floor in the '90s, I've had a sense of calm about my spirituality.

I fell deep into dance culture because I wanted that powerful connection with people *all the time.* I love sharing the joy of dance and celebrating with all walks of life. In dance culture, we are ALL family. Equality is something that was strongly promoted in early rave culture. Our code was "PLUR," which stood for Peace, Love, Unity, and Respect.

FRED: Beautiful. Martha Graham said, "Dance is the hidden language of the soul of the body." It sounds like you were in a family of soulful hippies!

LINDA: Indeed! A bunch of digital hippies! We took care of each other like family. In addition, processing of human emotion is totally allowed on the dance floor. It's not uncommon to see someone crying while dancing, or in their own world with their eyes closed. Dance is a powerful form of therapy, so it's OK to show emotion and work it out. I believe that the new generation of dancers, in modern-day EDM festival culture, adhere to many of these values as well.

Another important part of electronic music culture is honoring differences. Each person can dance differently, and that's OK! Each interpretation and movement style is valued by the group. It's like a potluck: if everyone brought salsa, it would be so boring, right?

FRED: It would be pretty damn boring, especially without my guacamole!

LINDA: Exactly! A great potluck happens when one person brings salsa, another a salad, someone brings dessert, and you'd bring your guacamole. The same goes for the dance floor. Everybody's unique contributions are encouraged and celebrated. That's part of my belief system as a teacher, as well.

After losing my friend in 2012, I left the underground scene and took my love of dance into the fitness world, away from the spiritual suffering of intoxicants. I was used to getting lost in free-form dancing, so it was a big transition at first. I had to go back to my roots in studio dance and learn to count steps, then lead others and cue steps ahead of time. I build the container; I have a playlist and I create basic movements, but I want people to deviate from that. I want them to let their freak flag fly. If they're off dancing in the corner by themselves, loving the process, I'm thrilled.

FRED: All about having the freedom of expression and flow.

LINDA: Exactly. Most people need a certain amount of guidance at first, but I like to remind them, over and over, that it's truly *their* dance, their body, and their spirit. More than anything, I love to get people high on movement. I love seeing people reach flow state.

When I feel down, stressed, or frustrated, dance helps me process and move those feelings into more productive energy. Part of my life's mission is to share this form of therapy. I love leading dance because I get to help people enhance their cardiovascular fitness, stimulate endorphins, and increase levels of BDNF (brain-derived neurotropic factor) for neuronal growth.

FRED: For many readers, BDNF may sound a little technical. But don't worry. I'm going to go into it more soon and give you further tips on boosting it. Please go on.

LINDA: That, from the physiological and spiritual standpoint, is how I'm guided these days to counter the world of unhealthy coping mechanisms, such as Big Tobacco. Rather than reaching for a cigarette, food, alcohol, or drugs, I want to help people seek out movement and dance. For this reason, I try to create an environment that is so much fun that it doesn't even feel like exercise.

FRED: With your science training and ongoing nursing education, what other tangible neurotransmitter (e.g., serotonin, dopamine, etc.) benefits do you sense in this fitness-based dance world?

LINDA: I'm not exactly sure. But I feel the social aspect, where we go around the room and connect with each other—similar to in the rave community—boosts the neurotransmitter oxytocin, and the "fitness as fun" aspect boosts two other neurotransmitters: dopamine and serotonin.

FRED: Research has shown that cardio workouts increase the brain-derived neurotropic factor (BDNF), which helps repair and regenerate neurons in our brain. This growth of new brain cells can improve memory and mood, and even reduce your risk of Alzheimer's.[182] In a sense, BDNF is like a "Miracle Gro" for your brain. (The stress hormone cortisol has the opposite effect.) So the combined effect of movement, music, socialization, and touch through dance further amplifies BDNF release. Additionally, as cortisol is reduced, there will be a reduction in inflammation, because dancing and music help release negative energies and bring in positive ones. Here's an expanded list of things that improve your BDNF levels:

- Exercise (especially, dance, interval exercise, resistance work)

- Sunshine

- Stress reduction (meditation, prayer)

- Quality sleep (test for sleep apnea, if you snore, or if you're overweight)

- Healthy, balanced organic diet with antioxidants from fruits like blueberries and pomegranate and with minimal intake of processed foods and sugars

- Maintenance of a healthy weight

- Balanced gut—consider testing your microbiome (bacterial balance in your stool) and if needed adding prebiotic foods and probiotics to optimize

- Balanced hormones (including thyroid, sex hormones, adrenal, and growth hormone)

- Intermittent fasting (ketogenic diet for even greater benefits)

- Curcumin, omega-3, resveratrol, coffee fruit, green tea

LINDA: There are many studies demonstrating the cognitive-enhancement properties of dance. It is—hands down—the absolute best exercise for preventing cognitive decline.

FRED: Indeed, and more fun than going to the gym!

LINDA: I believe that as long as humans have existed, we have cultivated joy, communicated stories, and celebrated life through dance. Dance is an important facet of cultural health, especially in these times. I like to embrace it and promote these primal aspects of being human.

FRED: I couldn't agree more. I feel that a lot of what's wrong in our society is this deprivation and deactivation of DNA in our deeper, more primal brain structures. So many of us are stuck in office spaces under fluorescent lights, staring at screens, becoming modern-day zombies, communicating through Facebook and Instagram instead of interacting more socially. Imagine how much better we'd all get along if we did more dancing, hiking, swimming in the ocean, and communed around a wilderness campfire under the stars. These primal needs are being replaced by technology, which I feel is often disruptive to our brain balance.

So, now that you've completed most of your prerequisites for nursing school, including genetics, do you feel that dancing, especially free-flowing, contributes to expressing healthier DNA, amplifying your spiritual self?

LINDA: There are many ways to look at it. I feel through dance I'm a lot more comfortable with myself. I believe that moving emotions through dance can help restructure neural networks. Replacing unhealthy coping mechanisms with healthier ones such as movement absolutely impacts our epigenetics.

Dance is a form of free therapy, and I'm very inspired to help other people find that, even if it's only a tiny bit of letting go at a time. Also, feeling connected to each other is perhaps one of the most important benefits epigenetically. The social aspects of dancing help me feel healthier and more willing to not only give, but receive love. I think that receiving is so much harder. I believe this has impacted my health and well-being in immeasurable ways. After turning to dance for so many years, I believe that my soul would be lost without this powerful form of therapy.

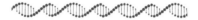

A Ballerina's Perspective

Sharon Wehner has been a principal ballerina at Colorado Ballet for over twenty years. She finished up her career in the 2017–'18 season with *Romeo and Juliet*. Given her spiritual pursuits and interests beyond the stage, she has a unique perspective on ballet.

FRED: I'd love to dive into your journey in dance, your spectacularly successful career, and your new life now as you leave the Colorado ballet. I'm interested in how dance may or may not have nurtured your spiritual self. Do you feel that you were able to expand and amplify this in your life during your years on stage?

SHARON: The thing about being a classical ballet dancer or even a modern dancer is that, on the one hand, you're still kind of a slave to the choreographer, choreography, directors, and the people who are telling you what to do. But that forces you to dance ever piece freshly, walking the tightrope between constraint and creativity.

Being at a certain level as a principal dancer, I've been allowed to express things—interpret passages. In general, I would say I most enjoyed the roles that tell a story, where the ballerina goes through a journey or a transformation and there is that permission to get into those extreme emotional places, explore those places. But now that that career is winding up, I want to be in the healing field: working with movement to allow people to express, release, or unlock things. The method I'm drawn to is called 5Rhythms®; it's a type of ecstatic therapeutic dance.

FRED: Yes, I've heard of it being done up in Boulder.

SHARON: They take you through five different types of music. Just free dancing—whatever comes up comes up. The first phase, you're connecting to your root chakra, so the cue is your feet on the floor. Then the next one is staccato, and the cue is more likely your hips—*move your pelvis*—so of course you're moving up through the chakras. Then they go into what's called chaos—which is pretty much driving techno music or anything that takes you out of your brain—and here you can work on anger and emotion. The idea is to move faster than you can think, because you're trying to bypass the cortex. Then come string instruments, such as cello, creating a calmer opening to the heart chakra. And since you hit chaos just before, you go back down the wave—allowing you to sob and release. It can be quite powerful. The last part is stillness, and that music brings you down on the ground.

FRED: Interesting, this flowing ecstatic type of dance guided by genres of music sounds. So therapeutic!

SHARON: Indeed. At one session a woman walked up to the facilitator, and the facilitator said, "Oh, I haven't seen you in a while." She replied, "Yeah, my brother just died this month"—very matter of fact. You could tell she was up in her head, very guarded—*my brother just died; it's been a lot*, blah, blah, blah. It was a very small group, and sure enough, once we got past the chaos and into the heart, it was super powerful. She was sobbing, and then we made this circle—dancing around her—for support. It was her way of getting into her heart. That's a different type of dance, where the structure might be giving cues, such as to use our arms as we work into the heart. Because in yoga, the main channel that goes through the heart is through your arms.

You can really perceive how the dance is helping people to connect and unlock a lot of things through a 5Rhythms sort of situation.

FRED: As a ballerina, do you sense when you are amplifying a certain chakra?

SHARON: Yes, but a lot of ballet dancers know nothing about the chakras. Because the tradition of ballet is so aesthetic, I think sometimes it can block that awareness; one of the big drawbacks of inexperienced dancers is that they can be so worried about how the position and the form look that they're not necessarily really feeling.

Ultimately I don't really dance for the aesthetics—it's not my motivation—but I'm in an art form that's very aesthetically focused.

FRED: How much natural flow can you get into within the boundaries of your role as principal ballerina?

SHARON: When you're working on something well, it's like turning the faucet on, and you feel like, *Oh yeah, this is like—God.* You can get there, certainly. And I think, like with anything, sometimes like in a yoga pose, if you're "off," it can be hurtful for your body, and flow is not going to be there in that case. There is something valid also about playing by the rules—in this case, knowing the technique backwards and forwards—in order to find the release.

FRED: When you look at classical ballet and how it's structured, how much freedom and creative unity are you able to express?

SHARON: I think it's a process. By the time you get on stage, we have a phrase, to *make it your own.* Hopefully, you've embodied that choreography, and then you're not fighting with it. It's *yours now.* It's when you're first learning choreography you're really up in your head. Sometimes I have to make up a story about this movement or that, and then it becomes more embodied.

FRED: Yes, we all have to adapt to the structured things that we don't necessarily enjoy. Unnecessary and excessive paperwork from my medical practice is something I fantasize about burning or blowing up daily!

SHARON: Yes, because that's part of the choreography.

FRED: How would you describe being "in the zone" in dance?

SHARON: For me a lot of it is about the music. It kind of flows through me. Sometimes I'll visualize Earth energy and the cosmic energy. It's again like turning on that faucet and flowing it through. That's what it feels like. If it's focused on character, then the flow really is the emotion, and the music that's flowing through is expressed through you, too.

FRED: Being in the flow with dance, work, or even making love is so vital to our happiness. I recently read in an article in the University of Colorado School of Medicine newsletter that you are using Gyrokinesis® to help patients with neurological disease.

SHARON: Yes, I teach dance to help those suffering from Parkinson's, and I'd love to expand that into dance for oncology patients.

In regard to Parkinson's patients, it bypasses some of their neurological blocks a bit. Having them move to music, it's really interesting to see how they transform, and once they have transformed, we give them a movement task while also feeling the music. It works different parts of the brain and helps improve balance and coordination. It even helps with their tremors and dystonia. It's pretty amazing how they might come in shuffling, but by the end of the class they're waltzing. How is it they can waltz across the floor, but not walk?

FRED: How are you stimulating the visual cortex?

SHARON: We use a lot of imagery; it's similar to a picture expressing a thousand words. The body can understand being a bird or being a leaf blown by the wind. Gyrokinesis is also focused on the spine, as we use circular and spiral movements to help open those. It feels dancy to people. We get their hips moving on stools, and then we go to some mat work. But yeah, you would be moving your hips; you would be moving your body, your arms in different planes too. Gyrokinetics is for anybody. People of all levels.

For me, I got into it because I wanted to work with this choreographer who was doing contemporary dance, and she told me she thought I was too locked into my classical training. After she recommended it, I did my first lesson. I remember we were doing some kind of twist and I just started crying. Something was unlocked as we did figure-eight forms, and I said, *Oh, my God, I feel like I'm going into the attic of my body.* I loved it.

FRED: If you were to pick one type of dance or movement that is more healing than others, which would it be?

SHARON: I think it's all up to the individual. Everybody has a dancer in them. People say, *I'm not a dancer*, or, *I don't know how to dance.* Are they referring to a particular style, such as ballroom? When I've gone to clubs, I've had people tease me. It's not my thing, but others can let loose and let go. I do really believe that everybody can connect with music and feel how it moves them, especially if they allow themselves to do it without judgment.

FRED: Lately, geneticists are finding that DNA may have a memory of sorts, not in such a way that mutation can be passed on to our children but more from an energetic level perhaps. I wonder if cultural dance skills can be epigenetically transferred to an individual, which can then be accessed more naturally than by somebody else, who didn't have that DNA imprinting by prior generations.

SHARON: I don't see why not; it's certainly evident in athletes.

FRED: Makes me laugh. I surely didn't pick up that gene! What types of movements do you feel are more activating spiritually?

SHARON: Various movements have their own unique flavors. So again, if one experiences the 5Rhythms type of dance, different movement will activate a different flavor in your body, and all of them are spiritual in a way, or emotional. Or they're just different, so they may tap into the unique flavors in your body. We're such multidimensional beings.

FRED: Do you feel that when you're dancing with a partner of the opposite sex, there's an element of masculine/feminine energy being generated that can amplify the field for you? Not necessarily in a sexual way, but in an energetic way?

SHARON: I think so. I think anytime you're dancing with someone, you have this sort of unspoken agreement about sharing space, sharing an energy field. It's a beautiful thing in itself—just human to human.

You know—coming back to the sexual piece—I have felt different energy sometimes, dancing with a gay partner, but not always. I think in classical ballet there's usually pretty clear gender roles. The man is supporting the woman, but not always. I've been told, especially when I first started dancing, that I'd have to *let him do it, let him do it, let him do it, don't lead him,* and that kind of thing. And then afterwards I might have to say, "You really had me off my leg here, and I am surrendering to that because that's my role, but it's uncomfortable." And then we'd have a discussion and hopefully next time he'd be OK. You know what I mean? It doesn't work if you're both in charge. So advancing is a microcosmic relationship.

FRED: Finding that balance between giving, receiving.

SHARON: Giving and taking or giving and receiving, and again I think it always works best when both people are listening to each other energetically and physically.

FRED: If sexual feelings did emerge with a fellow dancer, could it enhance the dance through a deeper, more primal energetic expression?

SHARON: Yes, it's something you have to learn. I think when you're younger, it's hard. Even eye contact is difficult. So when you learn as a professional, you can have intimacies but they don't really extend beyond that bubble of the dance.

FRED: Just like actors on the screen. From your intuitive perspective, do you feel people can change their DNA through dance and movement, shifting it in a favorable way?

SHARON: Intuitively, I'd say yes. Anything that you do that affects your biochemistry and your neurological signals and emotions will influence your cells.

FRED: Thank you so much for your perspective from your twenty years as principal ballerina at the Colorado Ballet. I can't wait to hear how you continue to transform others after you leave the stage later this season.

Neurological Benefits of Dance

From a broader perspective, dance—with its rapidly changing, challenging routines for the brain, its music, its spiritual and energetic balancing, and its social interaction—helps us stay young. Take the example of Dance for PD®. The Mark Morris Dance Group, together with the Brooklyn Parkinson Group, founded it in 2001. Now it's in over twenty-four countries. Thirty-eight peer-reviewed scientific studies have shown evidence of its effectiveness and benefits. Jay Baruch, MD (Associate Professor of Emergency Medicine, Alpert Medical School, Brown University), states: *"Dance for Parkinson's Disease is more than a possible therapy or treatment . . . it's a dose of meaningfulness for these patients. It's a small jewel that gets them working on something that helps them feel connected."*[183]

Dancing and the benefits to brain health warrant further research to determine which types of dance (and exercise) help regenerate and preserve brain function.

Exploring the regenerative, anti-aging aspects of exercise, a 2017 German study analyzed this by observing the size of the hippocampus—"an area that controls memory, learning and balance." It reported: "Knowing that aerobic, sensorimotor and cognitive training contribute to hippocampal volume, which also seems to be associated with balancing capabilities, we initialized a prospective, randomized longitudinal trial over a period of 18 months in healthy seniors. It concluded that both dance and endurance training 'can induce hippocampal plasticity in the elderly, but only dance training improved balance capabilities.'"[184]

From the abstract:

> Age-related degenerations in brain structure are associated with balance disturbances and cognitive impairments. However, neuroplasticity is known to be preserved throughout lifespan and physical training studies with seniors could reveal volume increases in the hippocampus (HC), a region crucial for memory consolidation, learning and navigation in space, which were related to improvements in aerobic fitness. Moreover, a positive correlation between left HC volume and balance performance

was observed. Dancing seems a promising intervention for both improving balance and brain structure
in the elderly.[185]

This difference is attributed to the extra challenge of learning
dancing routines."[186]

A widely cited earlier study, by the Albert Einstein College of
Medicine and the Department of Psychology and the Center for
Health and Behavior, Syracuse University *(New England Journal
of Medicine* 2001), with the title "Leisure Activities and the Risk
of Dementia in the Elderly,"[187] examined the relationship between
leisure activities and dementia in 469 participants between the ages
of seventy-five and eighty-five. It concluded that *"Participation in
leisure activities is associated with a reduced risk of dementia."*

From its evaluations, running over twenty-one years, it determined that "Among cognitive activities, reading, playing board
games, and playing musical instruments were associated with a
lower risk of dementia. Dancing was the *only physical* activity associated with a lower risk of dementia."

In "Use It or Lose It—Dancing Makes You Smarter Longer,"
Richard Powers, an instructor at Stanford University's Dance
Division who has taught social dances for over forty years, digs
deeper: "A major study added to the growing evidence that stimulating one's mind by dancing can ward off Alzheimer's disease
and other dementia, much as physical exercise can keep the body
fit. Dancing also increases cognitive acuity at all ages," he writes.

He summarized the twenty-one-year-long Albert Einstein College
research: "They . . . studied physical activities like playing tennis

or golf, swimming, bicycling, dancing, walking for exercise and doing housework." None, it turned out—with one exception—lent protection against dementia, despite having possible cardio-vascular benefits. "The only physical activity to offer protection against dementia was frequent dancing. . . . As Harvard Medical School psychiatrist Dr. Joseph Coyle explains in an accompanying commentary: 'The cerebral cortex and hippocampus, which are critical to these activities, are remarkably plastic, and they rewire themselves based upon their use.'"

Richard Powers elaborated, "More is better. *Do whatever you can to create new neural paths.* The opposite of this is taking the same old well-worn path over and over again, with habitual patterns of thinking and living." He drew on an aphorism of a young person walking on stepping stones across a creek:

> The focus of that aphorism was creative thinking, to find as many alternative paths as possible to a creative solution. But as we age, parallel processing becomes more critical. . . . Randomly dying brain cells are like stepping stones being removed one by one. Those who had only one well-worn path of stones are completely blocked when some are removed. But those who spent their lives trying different mental routes each time, creating a myriad of possible paths, still have several paths left.
>
> As the study shows, we need as many of those paths active as we can while also generating new paths, to maintain the complexity of our neuronal connections.
>
> In other words, *Intelligence—use it or lose it.*[188]

Later research is fine-tuning the conclusions; for example, partnership tango was more effective in one study than solitary dance. In general, positive results come from activities that best fit the injunction to keep the mind challenged. Subtleties with regard to any activity can aim for this goal of increasing the routes and "stepping stones" in the brain.

Potential Benefits of 3-D Video Games

Extrapolating from the above, not surprisingly, a reasonable amount of video gaming by older people (when compared with piano lessons) has also been found to improve memory and aids in resisting cognitive decline.

> In a small study published in the journal *PLOS* ONE [a primary-research journal of the Public Library of Science], researchers found that older adults who played 3D platform games, like Super Mario 64, had more gray matter within their hippocampus—an important region of the brain associated with memory—after playing the popular action-adventure game.
>
> "3D video games engage the hippocampus into creating a cognitive map, or a mental representation, of the virtual environment that the brain is exploring," study author Gregory West, an assistant psychology professor at the University of Montreal, said in a statement.[189]

Although I'm not an advocate for video games with violent content and am concerned about increased screen time and the inactivity it can create, leading to further rises in obesity, it is, however, interesting to note these favorable changes to the hippocampus. Our family used to enjoy Wii Fit with our kids in the mid-2000s, including Dance Revolution, We Ski, etc.—using the balance board and other accessories. This got us off the couch on rainy days, making exercise via visual stimulation and sound more fun. Recently, my wife and I purchased a Peloton stationary bike with high-definition videos (not 3-D yet) that also hopefully enhances hippocampus gray matter. We need further studies on guided meditations that visualize nature while at the same time supporting relaxation; and it would be helpful to have the results contrasted with the 3D-video-game impact on deep brain stimulation. This way, we can include those whose entry point to mindfulness and brain stimulation may only be through technology.

Yoga

Last but not least, the rise and continued popularity of yoga has had a powerful effect on movement, flexibility, and mindfulness. It offers easy access in metro-area studios, and for those living remotely it can be streamed to your screen. Yoga's origins are believed to date back at least to 600 BC, but likely further (Wikipedia). In 1893, in a powerful speech at the World Parliament of Religions in Chicago, Swami Vivekananda sparked interest in it. Later, in 1920, Paramahansa Yogananda promoted yoga to a large group of Boston progressives. Other forms, including the introduction of Kundalini yoga in 1969 by Yogi Bhajan, followed.[190] Then, in the 1980s, Dean Ornish amplified mainstream interest by promoting yoga's heart-health benefits. Another huge growth spurt occurred from 2001 to 2011, when the number of practitioners blossomed from 4 to 20 million. Sometime in the early '90s I began my practice and continue to enjoy it today. The postures and breathwork have always been powerfully helpful in strengthening, stretching, and relaxing me, especially when I do yoga outdoors. I often think that if I were a trust funder, I'd spend my mornings in yoga and afternoons skiing or biking. My busy practice doesn't quite allow that! Recently, I tried the new, trendy NIA workout at a local Denver studio. It combines elements of martial arts, yoga, and modern dance to all sorts of music, including electronica. To me it had an element of ecstatic dance, promoting an aerobic-like, fast-paced free flow. While I was the only guy in this group of twenty, I still had lots of fun trying to keep up with their more skillful and polished moves. Its popularity is growing fast here.

Regardless of the dance genre or meditative movement you enjoy, they all have unique benefits to your physical, emotional, and DNA health. Simply getting your body moving to music or postured into energetic flow is therapeutic. Being the adventurous type, I love spicing it up and taking myself out of my comfort zone at times. Will I try belly dancing at some point? Well, that one is stretching it!!! As Linda said, "Have fun, let your freak flag fly, and get into flow!"

Chapter 8

The Potential of Plant Medicine and Modern Derivatives to Open Your Mind and Enhance Your Genome

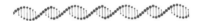

I n 2017, Dey Street Books published the national best seller *Stealing Fire: How Silicon Valley, the Navy SEALs, and Maverick Scientists Are Revolutionizing the Way We Live and Work* by Steven Kotler, a journalist, and Jamie Wheal, an expert on the neurophysiology of human performance. The two are the founders of the global Flow Genome Project, whose goal is, by 2020, to map the genome of Flow (peak performance state) and give universal free access to it.

They opened *Stealing Fire* in 415 BC, in a scene where ancient Greeks imbibed *kykeon*, a sacred elixir that brought them to higher spiritual states. Though very little is known about kykeon or what was actually drunk in the ancient Mysteries in the small town of Eleusis outside Athens, what is known—and what is the point of the book—is that the Mysteries were a time to get "out of the head," into a non-ordinary, or "altered," state of aware-ness. Many well-known people participated, as demonstrated by ancient writings. Kotler and Wheal speculate that Plato's concept of the sacred geometric forms was impacted by this ceremony; likewise, Pythagoras may have received insights on his music of the spheres concept in this way.[191] Czech psychiatrist Stanislav Grof, a pioneer in transpersonal psychology, in his foreword to *LSD: MY Problem Child*, goes as far if not further:

> People from our culture, who see the use of psyche-delic plants as something that is practiced in exotic and "primitive" cultures, and is alien to our tradition would be very surprised to find out that psychedelic substances very likely profoundly influenced the an-cient Greek culture, generally considered the cradle of the European civilization. Many giants of Greek culture, including Plato, Aristotle, Alkibiades, Pinda-ros, and others were initiates in the Mediterranean mysteries of death and rebirth held in the names of Demeter and Persephone, Dionysus, Attis, Adonis, Orpheus, and others.

Investigating peak brain performance, the *Stealing Fire* authors discovered that today, on a widespread basis—sometimes in se-cret—many highly successful Americans are pursuing eclectic "state-changing techniques," including various "kykeon" plant and fungi medicines. That might take the form of traditional plant medicines, LSD, neurofeedback, transcranial magnetic and electrical brain stimulation, meditation, and cardiac-coherence devices—to name some of the modern ways to achieve *ecstasis* (to "stand outside oneself and to be filled with inspiration").[192] This, they call "flipping the switch."

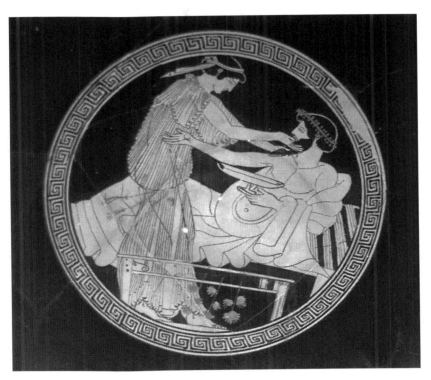

A Kykeon moment?

My Personal Journey

My journey to "flip the switch" began in shamanic circles later in life. When I was growing up, my parents took me to a fairly liberal Presbyterian church. While it was more open minded and never created a guilt-infused consciousness, as the Catholic and Baptist churches sometimes do, I wanted a purer connection to God—for example, through meditating and providing help to others, rather than listening to a filtered, secondhand version from the pulpit.

I had been ramping up my interest—dipping into shamanic books, studying Chinese medicine, qigong, etc.—since 1996. But in my early forties, out of the blue three patients in one week told me to *study* shamanism. No discussion of this preceded their statements, which I found both auspicious and synchronistic, motivating me to move from contemplation to action. To see if shamanism might be a good fit, I attended a weekend workshop run by a Michael Harner facilitator. Harner, author of the classic *Way of the Shaman*, had created the workshop. The weekend introduced me to the breadth of shamanism. Afterwards, I attended a workshop led by internationally acclaimed don Oscar Miro-Quesada, the originator of the Pachakuti Mesa Tradition: cross-cultural shamanism.

Motivated still further, I signed up for a year-long apprenticeship with his facilitators in monthly trainings in Boulder, where with twelve other participants, I experienced and learned about this high Andes Peruvian shamanism. One ritual I found particularly powerful was when, in a circle, using a "mesa," which is much like a small personal altar, we'd, one by one, meditatively integrate our faith—Christian, Buddhist, Muslim, Hindu, Jewish, etc.— into the cosmos and anchor it into Mother Earth (upper/middle/lower worlds) and ourselves.

This intense foundation, combined later with my guided exploration with plants with psychoactive properties, reconnected me to my inner self and God. As the teaching progressed, I became a better, more intuitive healer. Things became more synchronistic and life much more meaningful.

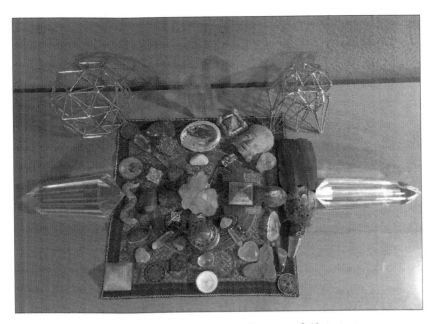

The author's "Mesa," containing elements of Christianity,
Buddhism, the Earth, and the cosmos

Studies and stories on how to get "out of the head"—into Flow,
into altered states—discussed by the *Stealing Fire* authors include
the practice of SEAL Team 6, who live or die depending on their
ability to precision-"merge" into one mind on a mission. They
do this through intense focus and intention. Mindfulness-based
tools figure in many success stories—among Fortune 500 execu-
tives, Wall Street traders, professional athletes, healthcare providers, participants at Google, and others. As wisdom teachers tell
us, we all have our own unique path. Finding what flows with you
and even feels timeless, as if you've been there before, will be the
best path forward.

Rocky Mountain Highs and the Potentials of Cannabis to Heal

It first occurred to me to include this controversial chapter when I found myself riding a quad chair at Breckenridge Ski Resort with snowboarders from Kansas. Most of my ideas come up during hikes, meditating, or in the shower, so this was different. As I sat in the chair, soaking up the scenery of lightly snow-covered pines, I looked over at them and thought: *Hmm, looks like college students up for a long weekend from out of state.* Not surprisingly, within a few minutes I found myself clouded in the smoke of our legalized and most popular Colorado herb. Looking to my right, I said, "I see you found more than one reason to come boarding here!" The guy responded, "Yes, we love this stuff" as he took another puff. "Connects us to nature and gets us in the flow as we carve up the mountain."

"Do you smoke it?" another asked.

"No," I replied, "I played with it here and there in college but never got much out of it. Perhaps since, like former President Bill Clinton, I never inhaled," I said with a wink.

"What!" he exclaimed. "You live in Colorado, where it's legal, and you don't smoke. Are you crazy?"

I replied, "Well, there are a lot of folks in Colorado that don't ski either! Now, those folks are crazy!" As we unloaded from the lift I wished them a fun and safe weekend of boarding.

Later as I relaxed at our mountain place, I contemplated whether or not to write this chapter. Wouldn't it be better to talk about something low risk like a gluten-free diet? Would conservative peers or medical societies I belong to criticize me for discussing this taboo topic? Would I have to defend it, by pointing out how many patients nationwide—perhaps in their own practice—died from inappropriate prescription of narcotics and other addictive, potentially lethal medications? Perhaps even reference the 2017 American Public Health Association article that showed—from 2000 to 2015 in Colorado—a 6.5 percent drop in opioid-linked deaths, believed to be due to the legalization of cannabis/marijuana. Are narcotic-pain patients who now use legal marijuana in Colorado finding some level of augmented pain relief, decreased anxiety, or even better sleep that allows them to decrease their use or dependency? This question has yet to be answered, but after hearing many of my patients speak candidly, I would say yes.

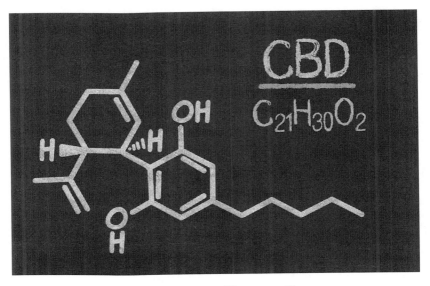

CBD structure (Shutterstock)

As a physician I have a great number of patients who confide in me about the benefits of recreational, spiritual, and medicinal marijuana. Some seek the high, while others use it to deepen their meditation. Many seek to relieve joint or muscle pain, insomnia, anxiety, depression, or other conditions they're struggling to alleviate with mainstream medical therapies. There is a big distinction between CBD (cannabidiol)—the non-psychoactive component of cannabis that can reduce inflammation and pain—most frequently used in medical marijuana, and THC, the psychoactive component that makes one high.

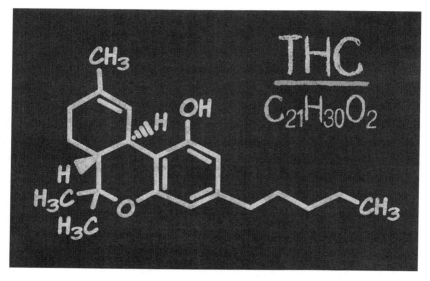

THC Structure (Shutterstock)

New to my practice, one desperate family relocated to Colorado primarily for access to the "Charlotte's Web" hemp strain to treat their son's seizure disorder. Traditional treatments were ineffective, so when they found this helped but wasn't available in their home state, they moved. This strain, which is high in cannabidiol, or CBD, and low (less than 0.3 percent) in the psychoactive THC oil, was developed by Stanley Brothers from hemp in 2011. Early results were inconclusive. But in 2017 Orrin Devinsky et al. reported in the *New England Journal* that "the percentage of patients who had at least 50 percent reduction in convulsive-seizure frequency was

43 percent with cannabidiol, and 27 percent with placebo."[193] The number of children now using it worldwide is in the millions.[194]

Moving to THC (tetrahydrocannabinol), the psychoactive component in cannabis, in 2016, the famed Salk Institute reported: CANNABINOIDS REMOVE PLAQUE-FORMING ALZHEIMER'S PROTEINS FROM BRAIN CELLS: "Preliminary lab studies at the Salk Institute find THC reduces beta amyloid proteins in human neurons." It elaborated:

> While these exploratory studies were conducted in neurons grown in the laboratory, they may offer insight into the role of inflammation in Alzheimer's disease and could provide clues to developing novel therapeutics for the disorder.
>
> "Although other studies have offered evidence that cannabinoids might be neuroprotective against the symptoms of Alzheimer's, we believe our study is the first to demonstrate that cannabinoids affect both inflammation and amyloid beta accumulation [plaque] in nerve cells," says Salk Professor David Schubert, the senior author of the paper.[195]

The next step would be a clinical trial.

Sanjay Gupta, MD, discusses the pain and anti-inflammatory benefits of marijuana in his April 2018 documentary, *Weed 4*. He states that 115 Americans die every day from opioid overdoses, and 2.5 million are currently struggling with opioid addiction. He interviewed Mike James, former NFL Tampa Bay Buccaneers running back, whose physician gave him a cocktail of opiates to manage the pain from an ankle fracture and surgery. Mike said, "I became immune to painkillers. Like I still had pain, and now I'm sedated, with pain." When Mike tried pot instead of pills in 2014, he experienced relief and mental coherence. He disagrees that marijuana is a gateway to drugs—and feels that football was his gateway to drugs, thanks to docs who prescribed them to help him stay in the game.

Mark Wallace, MD, director of the Pain Medicine Center at the University of California, San Diego, told Dr. Gupta, "We were taught in medical school to prescribe opioids . . . and told that there's evidence that opiates are probably not that risky and that we should use them more liberally." In 1999 Dr. Wallace and others received a share of a 10 million-dollar California state grant to study cannabis as an alternative to opioids. Using pot, 80 percent of his patients—hundreds of them—were weaned off pills.

While I am in no way a "weed doc," I provide several physician certifications a year for medical marijuana, consistent with Colorado legal and medical requirements. To help reduce inflammation and pain, I also frequently recommend CBD (THC free) oil to patients and have seen amazing results.

According to Dr. Gupta, no one has ever died from a marijuana overdose, and he sees cannabis as a potential gateway to recovery—getting off narcotics and feeling better.[196]

In fact, other psychoactive plants, not discussed by Dr. Gupta—such as ayahuasca and the controversial ibogaine—are showing promise to clear patients of narcotic and alcohol addiction. Ayahuasca is considered a safer treatment than ibogaine, which can have adverse effects on heart electrical conduction. Both need further research and appropriate professional medical screening/administration in the countries where they are legal. The Multidisciplinary Association for Psychedelic Studies (MAPS) has supported studies on both, with encouraging results.[197] Larger-scale longer-term studies are needed to determine efficacy. In the future, I would like to see research that collects data to correlate subjects' QEEG Brain mapping, functional brain imaging (fMRI, SPECT) and heart rate variability while using these plants.

Our country is suffering from an out-of-control opioid crisis, thanks to prescribing habits of "pain clinics," urgent care centers, ERs, and providers who are reaching for narcotics inappropriately to break a migraine, reduce back pain, and other pain-related issues that can frequently be treated alternatively, with an NSAID (ibuprofen-like compounds). Perhaps narcotic prescribing gets these facilities more glowing Yelp reviews, while shortening the visit, due to this win (marketing)/win (financial) incentive. According to the CDC, 70,200 Americans died from drug overdoses in 2017, the majority from narcotics, 17,000 of which were prescribed.[198] The CDC and other organizations have responded to this crisis by enacting stricter guidelines and oversight to help reduce the inappropriate prescribing of narcotics. Despite this and more addiction-center funding, we still have a long way to go. Again, a more integrative, proactive approach might have saved many lives up front.

Additionally, excess consumption of alcohol was responsible for "approximately 88,000 deaths and 2.5 million years of potential life lost (YPLL) each year in the United States 2006–2010." This equates to an average shortening of their life span by thirty years.[199]

When one looks simply at annual morbidity from narcotics, alcohol and tobacco, it becomes obvious that the government has been strongly influenced by lobbying efforts of these industries. The latest strategy by the tobacco industry to get youth addicted to nicotine for life and maintain profits is though e-cigarettes. The CDC stats (for 2018) show that 20.8 percent of high school students and 4.9 percent of middle-schoolers are using them. Compared to 2017, that's an alarming 78 percent increase in high schoolers, and 48 percent increase in middle-schoolers—amounting to 3.6 million middle and high school students using e-cigs. Combine that with childhood obesity, and this is a cardiovascular crisis in the making, not to mention DNA damage. Are Congress and our surgeon general doing enough to abate this?[200]

Don't even get me started on the gun lobby, resulting in thousands of deaths annually incurred in our country! Research internationally has shown which substances have the greatest abuse potential and risk of death. This chart (below) from a Lancet study—where alcohol, heroin, and crack cocaine are at the top—summarizes it best.[201] Remember that most heroin addiction begins with prescribed narcotic use: "A study of young, urban injection drug users interviewed in 2008 and 2009 found that 86 percent had used opioid pain relievers nonmedically prior to using heroin."[202] Unfortunately, the chart does not include prescribed narcotics, which would be right next to alcohol.

Quite clearly, the legal availability of many of the most harmful substances and the restriction of others has been influenced by lobbyists and politicians, rather than by looking at the big realistic picture of what is harmful and lethal public health. Most of us know someone killed by a drunk driver; every night on the news we are informed of such tragic deaths. Have you ever heard of someone being killed enjoying a psilocybin-mushroom journey? Contemplating the reality of harm from what our country has deemed legal and safe versus what was outlawed for political reasons motivated me to shed light on this important subject.

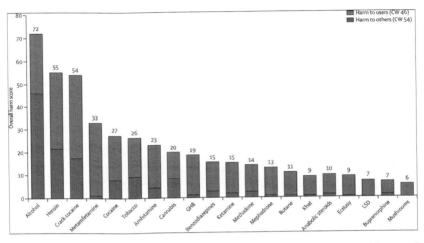

This bar graph from a Lancet study demonstrates the high potential harm of alcohol and tobacco, compared to very low risk from psilocybin and psychedelics at the far right. Source: https://www.thelancet.com/journals/lancet/article/PIIS0140-6736(10)61462-6/fulltext.

Using Psychoactive Plant Medicines to Heal. Why did the ancient Greeks and many others use "kykeon" and other plant medicines?

Let's take a step back in time to the ancient indigenous cultures that used these plants for hundreds of years—calling them "medicines." They are not for recreation. The relationship of indigenous cultures with the plants was entirely different from our Western relationship to medicines.

A "Historical Review of Traditional Plants' Usage" in *Pharmacognosy Review* begins: "Healing with medicinal plants is as old as mankind itself. . . . Awareness of medicinal plants' usage is a result of the many years of struggles against illnesses due to which man learned to pursue drugs in barks, seeds, fruit bodies, and other parts of the plants." Gradually, there was a move away from this relationship with plants so important to our forefathers:

> Ever since ancient times, in search for rescue [from] their disease, the people looked for drugs in nature. The beginnings of the medicinal plants' use were instinctive, as is the case with animals. In view of the fact that at the time there was not sufficient information either concerning the reasons for the illnesses or concerning which plant and how it could be utilized as a cure, everything was based on experience. In time, the reasons for the usage of specific medicinal plants for treatment of certain diseases were being discovered; thus, the medicinal plants' usage gradually abandoned the empiric framework and became founded on explicatory facts. Until the advent of iatrochemistry [medical chemistry] in [the] 16th century, plants had been the source of treatment and prophylaxis. Nonetheless, the decreasing efficacy of synthetic drugs and the increasing contraindications of their usage make the usage of natural drugs topical again.[203]

The ancients used plants to heal, to expand consciousness, and to learn. One plant or combination of plants can address different levels of a condition—simultaneously working the physical, emotional, and energy body. Sometimes plants root out an emotional block; or, they amplify a sense of community or connectedness with the universe, and have even been documented to have healed a life-threatening illness. Other times they may induce a vision of how to solve a problem. According to shamans, while talking to the medicines they activate them, adding healing intentions, particularly in brewing ayahuasca and San Pedro. As the shapibo shamans of the Amazon sing "icaros," the plant is guided though the bodies of those drinking it ceremonially; this produces deeper healing. Indigenous tribal shamans from around the world may likewise sing or chant messages.

Using psychoactive plants in this way may be similar to the respect given to wine during communion, as opposed to getting drunk at a wine-tasting bar. Likewise, one can consume them with respect and the intention to be healed and spiritually transformed or, by contrast, simply do it to get high. In Peru for example, foreigners visit the rainforest to experience the Shipibo "sacrament," ayahuasca. Luckily, many centers are now performing more rigorous screening:

> Omar Gomez, from the Rainforest Healing Center, says he turns away 60% of potential visitors: either because they have problems that ayahuasca doesn't mix with (such as schizophrenia) or because they're not sufficiently serious about it.
>
> "We do an intense screening process to make sure we don't have any psychedelic tourists," says Gomez. "Right now the ayahuasca industry is booming. But we want to make sure that the people who come are people that have a strong intention and desire to heal."[204]

Psychoactive plants may ultimately present a powerful tool in shifting our thoughts away from habitual thinking. The older we get, the more vulnerable we become to preconditioning, as neural tracts become ingrained in various regions of our brain, from our cortex to our deep brain structures (i.e., hippocampus, amygdala). The psychoactive plants may stimulate diverse neural connections, reaching beyond the familiar pathways. This can increase creativity and the inner knowing of our unconscious to assist in healing our bodies and mind.

The experience may also improve well-being and enhance our genome, while making us less egocentric and more present with others and ourselves.

Advanced civilizations of the past, as well as many contemporary indigenous tribes, sought or seek enlightenment. Why are we obstructing an individual's potential for further spiritual growth by making them illegal, when there are few, if any, documented annual deaths? It is alarming that our society is not motivated into seeking solutions to help reduce the loss of eighty-eight thousand Americans from alcohol-related causes annually, of which close to 10 percent are innocent victims of drunk drivers.[205]

Even more concerning are the weak penalties for drunk driving. This is contrary to any public healthcare logic, simply statistics-wise, and clearly due to politics and the alcohol lobby. Deaths related to guns and tobacco, and their ongoing protection from paid-off politicians, has allowed this health crisis to accelerate as well. Yet, plant medicines, such as psilocybin, are not legal, and studies have clearly shown them to carry a small fraction of the risk that alcohol presents. Furthermore, narcotic use, most of which is prescribed, cost our country 218,000 lives from 1999 to 2017; that's a fivefold increase in 2017 compared to 1999. It wasn't until 2018 that the alarms were sounded to physicians and the public on this epidemic. Are we blind to this reality or just slow to wake up?

Let's talk about consciousness. The Irish Association of Humanistic and Integrative Psychotherapy and Psychology website describes everyday consciousness versus non-ordinary:

> Our normal, everyday state-of-consciousness, domi-
> nated by the ego, can be called "ordinary reality," and
> all other realms of the psyche or states-of-conscious-
> ness can be called "non-ordinary." In a non-ordinary
> state of consciousness, the universe can appear fluid
> and non-mechanical, space and time are relative,
> moral absolutes vanish, death is but a transition and
> life exists in a variety of forms. Stanislav Grof, one
> of the world's foremost researchers into the healing
> properties of non-ordinary states of consciousness,
> calls ordinary reality "hylotropic," meaning matter-
> orientated, and the latter, non-ordinary reality, "holo-
> tropic," meaning wholeness-orientated.[206]

Perhaps it is our individual or cultural departure from experiencing ecstasy and non-ordinary states of consciousness that is leading us down a narrow field of awareness more focused on materialism, ego, and technology.

Javier Regueiro, in *San Pedro Huachuma: Opening the Pathways of the Heart*, has a useful description: "Spiritual practices, as well as the plant medicine path, are not substitutes for life, but tools to help us engage with our lives, and the life of this planet with more clarity and lightness of being."[207] Plant medicine "is an uncovering and rediscovering of the seeds of wisdom we call carry within ourselves since the beginning of creation."[208]

Javier says, with proper usage they "help us become more aware that we are part of the greater whole, they open the ways for a different relationship with the Earth and all of its inhabitants."[209]

In a study for his PhD dissertation in Religion and Society at Harvard in 1962, Walter Pahnke, later MD, had Timothy Leary and Richard Alpert as advisors in what became famously known as the Marsh Chapel experiment, or "Miracle of Marsh Chapel."[210] The idea was to test whether a genuine religious experience of lasting impact would be facilitated in a Good Friday service if a hallucinogenic plant was taken just beforehand. Their results were quite positive and I will go into them extensively below, at the time of follow-up studies, forty years later.

Venture capitalist Tim Ferriss, # 1 *New York Times*, *Wall Street Journal* best-selling author of *The 4-Hour Workweek*, reports that opening the mind through psychoactive plants is common these days in unexpected quarters, even mainstream corporate America: "Once Steve Jobs and other successful people began recommending the use of psychedelics for enhancing creativity and problem solving, the public became more open to the possibility." On CNN he added, "The billionaires I know, almost without exception, use hallucinogens on a regular basis. [They're] trying to be very disruptive and look at the problems in the world . . . and ask completely new questions."

The *Stealing Fire* website calls flow "the state north of happiness," where everything flows magically, as when the athlete is "in the zone." Or a yogi is deep in meditation. They also call it rather humorously "mystical states on tap."[211] While some execs choose to attend a Tony Robbins motivational seminar, others, wanting a deep dive, travel to Central and South America to journey with shamans and the medicines. Hugely significant boosts in creativity, learning, and productivity were the outcome of using flow techniques, including the psychedelics.

Can Westerners, including entrepreneurs, participate respectfully in a sacred circle with shamans and their medicine? If the primary intention is self-healing and stimulation of creativity, compassion, etc., then I feel it still honors the sacredness of these plants and the shamans administering them.

The History of Plant Medicine Legalities in the United States

Why did the U.S. government block access to these plants and substances in 1970? The heinous reality of the Vietnam War in the '60's was difficult to process for most conscious and compassionate people. Watching the daily body counts of lost family and friends on TV, recognizing it was a war we never should have entered, created two primary ways to mitigate the emotional pain—by nationwide protest and/or by escapism. However, both were despised and/or feared by the government: 1) expression of anti-Vietnam War sentiment though the protest movement resulted in tragedy at Kent State University and elsewhere, and 2) the hippy movement, which embraced love and transcendental states of mind to further counter reality of their loved ones being killed in war, attracted government fear and hostility as well. In the backlash that ensued, LSD, mushrooms, and other entheogens became illegal. In my opinion, this was a foolish knee jerk reaction by Congress.

> In 1962, the U.S. Congress passed new drug safety regulations, and the Food and Drug Administration designated LSD as an experimental drug and began to clamp down on research into its effects. The following year, LSD hit the streets in the form of liquid soaked onto sugar cubes; its popularity grew quickly and the hippy counterculture was in full swing by the summer of 1967.[212]

The result was the Controlled Substances Act (CSA), Title II of the Comprehensive Drug Abuse Prevention and Control Act of 1970, banning this class and other potentially therapeutic compounds.

An unintended side effect, I believe, was that many more lives were lost to alcohol, tobacco, heroin, and other narcotics—as a more accessible alternative. Interestingly enough, we are finding that psychoactive plants, such as ayahuasca (a vine from the Amazon), have been more successful in breaking drug and alcohol addiction than traditional abstinence programs. According to acclaimed addiction specialist Dr. Lance Dodes, author of *The Sober Truth: Debunking the Bad Science Behind 12-Step Programs and the Rehab Industry*, traditional 12-step programs such as AA have a very low success rate—of only 5–10 percent.[213]

Some of the most powerful plant medications are ayahuasca, San Pedro, peyote, psilocybin, DMT, and 5-MeO-DMT derived from the dried venom of the Sonoran Desert toad, Bufo alvarius.

All except laboratory-synthesized DMT have been used by cultures indigenous to the Americas. After hard-fought battles by American Indians, Congress legalized the nondrug use of peyote in religious ceremonies by the Native American Church with passage of the Religious Freedom Restoration Act in 1993. In 2006 the U.S. Supreme Court unanimously ruled that the Brazilian-founded UDV church could use ayahuasca for religious purposes. This exemption would extend to the Santo Diame Church.[214] Likewise, to the Native American Church (peyote), União do Vegetal and Church of the Holy Light of the Queen (ayahuasca) and, to a lesser extent, Rastafarians (cannabis). More ayahuasca churches are springing up, in the U.S. Except for hemp-derived cannabidiol, U.S. law on the whole does not recognize medicinal use of psychoactive plants.

Over the next decade, I am hopeful that the Multidisciplinary Association for Psychedelic Studies (MAPS) and other organizations and individuals can successfully advocate for a legal, safe reintroduction of these psychoactive plants.

The Dark Side of Big Pharma

Like many industries, the pharmaceutical industry has a light and dark side to their business. I am thankful to medications for the many patients I've seen saved from infections, heart attacks, diabetic ketoacidosis, inflammatory and immunologic conditions, cancer, and more. But I also mourn the deaths of patients who have died from allergic reactions, drug resistance, narcotic overdose, and accidents under the influence of certain medications. I'd like to share my perspective as a quarterback in our broken system. My apologies for having to get this off my chest. It's a short digression!

I've been practicing in primary care twenty-six years now, and find it concerning that providers and the general public believe that drug therapy is the first line therapy for virtually everything. It really is easier in our modern world to prescribe medications, than to make an effort to treat the underlying condition more naturally. The pharmaceutical industry influences providers' prescribing habits beginning in medical school, PA school, and nursing school and continues to do so throughout our entire career as they sponsor meetings and lunches and place ads in all the journals we read. It's much easier to remember a drug name for depression and electronically prescribe an antidepressant with a click, than discuss psychotherapy, mindfulness, and stress reduction in a ten-minute visit.

My biggest concerns pertain to the overprescribing or inappropriate prescribing of psychotropics (antidepressants, antianxiety meds, and mood stabilizers) and narcotic medication classes that need greater research on safety and efficacy.

For example, the use of antidepressants has soared over the last decade, yet suicide rates, homicides, and mass shootings have continued to climb. In 2016, the U.S. suicide rates reached 44,965, up another 2,100 from 2014. (From the WISQARS Fatal injury Report—CDC. Suicide Injury Deaths and Rates per 100,000. All Races, Both Sexes, All Ages.)[215]

The five-year increase in suicides from 1999 to 2014 was very worrisome, at 24 percent, and we have yet to get stats for 2018 and beyond.[216] Many suicides go unreported; it is the second leading cause of death for young people aged fifteen–twenty-four.[217]

I attribute six primary causes to climbing numbers of suicides:

1. In most studies, antidepressants have been shown to be minimally effective, rarely beyond the benefit of a placebo except in severe depression.[218] (Sad, but true.)

2. While some have improved, I have witnessed many of my patients becoming blunted, not caring about any-thing—listless, losing passion—after starting these medications. It's easier to take your life when you feel blunted and don't give a flip. It's called "disrupted in-teroception." More on this soon.

3. Antidepressants have numerous side effects, includ-ing the black-box warning of "may increase risk of suicidality." What's equally worrisome is that some studies show it "may increase the risk of homicidality." Additional adverse effects include agitation, anxiety, insomnia, nausea, lethargy, sexual dysfunction, head-ache, and dizziness.[219] In a 2016 systematic review of antidepressants used in double blinded, placebo-controlled trials of healthy adults, the researchers dis-covered that antidepressants double the occurrence of events that lead to suicide and violence. Treating just sixteen patients with antidepressants leads to at least one of them being at risk for suicide or violence (95 percent confidence interval, 8 to 100).[220] The Na-tional Institute on Drug Abuse reported 5,269 Ameri-can deaths due to antidepressant overdoses in 2017.[221] A simple review of the literature and gun mortality in the United States clearly shows that easy access to

guns (while starting an antidepressant that has these potential side effects) is a dangerous cocktail. Does it not worry you that there are thousands of folks who own guns, drink alcohol daily, and are on antidepressants?? In fact, over one half of all suicides occur by firearms. Which leads me to #4.

4. Easy access to guns. The NRA wants you to believe that guns protect you, while the reality is in 2017 there were 15,633 gun-related deaths in our country.[222] While one assumes the government really cares about public health, it's hard to reconcile that with their inability to assist in effective gun-control legislation, regardless of the Second Amendment challenges. Another black-box warning for guns is needed: "Possession of a gun is statistically proven to improve the efficacy of your suicide, or is more likely to be used in homicidal action towards family members or others rather than in self-defense." So how many guns are "on the record" in our country? "U.S. civilians alone account for 393 million (about 46 percent) of the worldwide total of civilian held firearms." This amounts to "120.5 firearms for every 100 residents."[223] That doesn't make me feel safer. Does it make you feel safer?

5. Insurance covers mental-health counseling poorly—reimbursing providers inadequately, and limiting the number of visits. Oftentimes, in view of the limited number of mental-health care professionals and crisis centers, no visit is available. Typically, medication is the primary Band-Aid. A Google search of "reim-

bursement in mental health" in 2018 produced 20.3 million results, which means, to me, there are not nearly enough options and resources for providers or patients to get the help they need.

6. Impact of social media and its stressful effect on self-image; the cruel act of bullying impacts children and adults. Look at President's Trump's tweets, and we can see how this bullying behavior is being modeled from the top. Recently, NBC News had a discussion on social media's possible contribution to the rising teen-suicide rate.[224] The social media impact is further compounded by easy access and addiction to smart-phones, facilitating antisocial behavior in public and private and trending us towards texting and taking selfies, rather than interacting with one another.

As we overmedicate with antidepressants, mood stabilizers, benzodiazepines (anxiety medication), and narcotics, rather than assisting individuals more holistically to heal themselves through talk therapy (psychotherapy), acupuncture, transcranial magnetic therapy, and many other natural therapies, we will continue to see suicide and homicide rates climb.

Eric Harris, who assisted with Dylan Klebold when they murdered thirteen fellow students at Columbine High school in 1999, south of my home, and then both committed suicide, was on a selective serotonin reuptake inhibitor (SSRI), a type of drug commonly prescribed to treat depression. The most frequently used antidepressants are serotonin reuptake inhibitors. These act by blocking the reuptake of serotonin at the presynapse of a neuron, thus making more serotonin available at the postsynaptic receptor.[225] I will come back to this further on in the chapter.

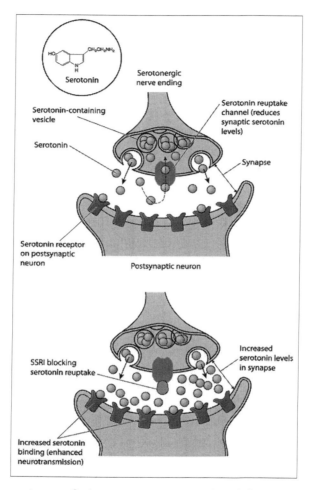

**Action of selective serotonin reuptake inhibitors
(SSRIs) at the synapse (Shutterstock)**

How many school shooters have been or will be shooting our innocent children as we fail to address the root cause of their depression, which often becomes agitated. The knee-jerk response to write a quick prescription for Prozac or its cousins can be harmful if one hasn't already addressed root cause through sufficient ongoing psychological, social, and family support. This deeper emotional support may prevent the disregard of their life, or others'.

Let me be clear. SSRIs don't make everyone agitated—or lose compassion and want to go out and shoot up a school or put a gun to their head. Sometimes they can help with depression, and more so with anxiety. However, if they are prescribed, ongoing support—along with close screening for adverse reactions of homicidality and violent thoughts, not just suicidality—should be performed. Ask if they have a gun in the house. And if a potential threat exists, notify agencies, as required by some state and federal laws, to block their purchase of guns. Also, providers should not cave to the life-threatening NRA opinion that "it's not a doctor's job to ask if there is a gun in the house"!!

To the east of me in Aurora, James Holmes, also under psychiatric care and on psychotropic medications, murdered twelve theatergoers, wounding many more, with his assault weapons. It would be interesting to know if adequate screening for violent behavior and preventative measures against gun access were made in his case.

Most recently, in 2018, our nation witnessed yet another horrific murder scene, in which Nikolas Cruz killed seventeen at the Parkland, Florida, high school. Will it ever end, and will our legislators and public wake up? These days, I see many patients walking in the door who are on four, sometimes five psychotropics. (Psychotropics are mood-altering medications.) Instead of a single med, many pharmaceuticals are now designed as "me too" medications to add onto an antidepressant that isn't effectively reducing depression, rather than stopping an ineffective one and trying another class.

The risk of adverse effects escalates with polypharmacy (multiple medications), as the recipients display obvious slowed cognitive function, and a zombie-like demeanor, or scientifically termed "disrupted interoception. What is interoception? A 2019 *Scientific American* article summarizes it well: "This lack of connection to our bodies can be looked at through a concept called interoception, which describes our awareness of internal bodily signals, including the detection of sensations such as hunger, thirst and heartbeat. Interoception is a process by which our brains/minds make sense of these signals, which serve as a running commentary or mental map of the body's internal world across conscious and unconscious levels of perception."[226] We've Lost Touch with Our Bodies but we can get it back through a process known as "interoception." In addition to drugs, our addiction to technology is also hacking into our interoception.

I help patients regain their sense of "aliveness" and interoception by safely and slowly tapering them off as many of these meds as possible, transitioning them to mindfulness-based activities such as breathwork, meditation, sound therapy, exercise, improved diet, and hormone balancing. (A sledge hammer to their phone would be a nice addition too!) This allows many to completely come off meds. It can take months, but typically a condition such as depression has been present in them for years. If needed, I can always restart medications, and I always encourage them to work with a therapist and/or a psychiatrist when needed.

The Impact of Big Pharma Greed

Let's also consider the impact of an overwhelming amount of pharmaceutical ads bombarding your brain via TV, radio, internet, social media, and print advertisements throughout your life. How has this affected your decision-making when it comes to addressing your health? The number of direct-to-consumer drug ads has grown astronomically. There's no need to reference an article or quote numbers here; simply turn on the evening news and count the number of drug ads you see in thirty minutes. They are telling you to ask your doctor about this drug or that, most of which cost ten thousand or more a month. Try Googling the cost of any medication advertised on TV, and you'll see why this is the medication they want you to take for life. It's quite enlightening and will give you an idea why they have plenty of money to lobby your legislators.

My personal research looking up the cost of drugs in ads run during the evening news showed the price typically 3–10 grand a month. No, the cost of medications is not simply research; it's also lobbying, marketing, and big profits. Drug companies typically price a new product high, then increase the price annually by 6 percent or more, not because they need to, but because they can. As noted in the chart, more than 5 billion annually is spent in direct-to-consumer marketing!

There seems to be no ethical consideration on affordability to the masses, and there are no legal limits on profiting 4,000 percent or more on a prescription for treating your medical condition.[227] Only the outrageous cost increase of the EpiPen caught the attention of Congress recently. More recently, Firdapse, a drug that treats Lambert-Eaton myasthenic syndrome, went from being free to being priced at $375,000 a year!!!! Why? Because a greedy company, Catalyst Pharmaceuticals, bought rights to it from the family-run Jacobus, then got FDA approval, repackaged it, and simply decided they wanted to make $375,000 on it annually off patients and our system because they can!![228] Not the best advertisement for American capitalism! Our U.S. healthcare system has no issue with placing profit over patient care and screwing us financially. Be sure to ask your legislators why meds in the U.S. are typically four times higher than in Canada, followed by asking how much money they accepted in campaign contributions from pharmaceutical companies.

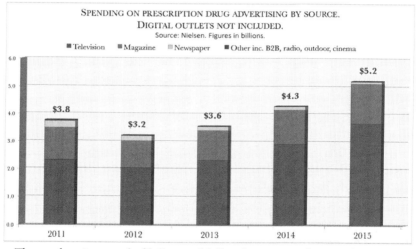

The accelerating trend of billions of dollars being spent by Big Pharma on direct-to-consumer marketing. Stat: Natalia Bronshtein.

Many medications are helpful and life-saving, and I still prescribe them, but I do so appropriately—only when it is the best option. Patients should beware of docs who have free-medication sample cabinets for this reason. Many prescriptions are harmful and life-threatening, such as Vioxx for arthritis (an anti-inflammatory Cox 2 inhibitor), which was pulled in 2004 after it was found to be causing fatal heart attacks and strokes. Who knows how many patients were started on this prescription via a free sample from the Vioxx rep! David Graham of the FDA made a conservative estimate of 60,000 lives lost from this drug. Yes, that's more than we lost in the Vietnam War.[229]

Natural Alternatives to Pharmaceuticals

Why not use a safer natural alternative such as turmeric (containing curcuminoids), rather than a cousin of Vioxx? It's effective for the treatment of arthritis when the curcumin compound is isolated and concentrated to 75 percent or higher into a capsule or pill. Because of its multitude of anti-inflammatory effects, this compound may also be helpful in the prevention of cancer, Alzheimer's, and other inflammatory diseases. Just think how many lives would have been saved if physicians had recommended perhaps a combination of curcumin, Tylenol, CBD oil, and acupuncture instead of Vioxx, or even Aleve. Finding the integrative approach for pain relief should be the direction, rather than using the latest expensive single-drug therapy left in a doc's drug-sample closet. Regarding the multitude of benefits from curcumin, see this review article—"Therapeutic Roles of Curcumin: Lessons Learned from Clinical Trials"—published by the National Institute of Health.[230]

In addition to curcumin, other amazing anti-inflammatory compounds include Omega-3 and pomegranate. Omega-3s are found in chia, flax, and coldwater fish such as salmon.[231]

Pomegranate juice and seeds can reduce your risk of heart disease by reducing plaque buildup in your coronaries (heart vessels), thanks to the high content of polyphenols, tannins, and anthocyanins.[232]

There are many other plants high in polyphenols, such as blueberries, dark chocolate, coffee, green tea, and pinot grapes. For a great review of these and other antioxidants that are powerful for your brain and body, read *Power Up Your Brain* by my fellow functional-medicine colleague David Perlmutter, M.D., with psychologist, medical anthropologist, author Alberto Villoldo, founder of the Four Winds Society and Light Body School. In my opinion, optimal brain health requires a strong nutritional foundation, with an organic diet including plant-based antioxidants, healthy fats (such as coconut oil, omega-3, monosaturated fats), B-complex vitamins, and vitamin D3. A healthy balanced gut/microbiome is also critical. I also encourage mindfulness-based therapies (as discussed in this book) and of course exercise.

Big Pharma Lobbies against Natural Therapies to Fight Competition!

As you are well aware, many politicians get endless donations from multibillion-dollar pharmaceutical companies lobbying for legislation and instilling bias favorable to new and existing drugs, and ignoring rising drug prices. Why do they also promote legislation against natural supplements, bioidentical hormones, and stem cell therapies? Simple. Because drug-company lobbyists financially back them, and assist them in introducing legislation to block competition from natural therapies.

We witnessed the latest unethical favoritism by President Trump in July 2018, when his administration blocked the introduction of a popular international resolution by Ecuador supporting breastfeeding—favoring instead the 70 billion-dollar infant-formula industry.[233] Why would one do this for anything other than financial favors from this industry?

Natural breast milk supports the best brain development in infants, aids in gut health (gut microbiome), reduces infant infection, psychologically helps bond the infant to Mom, reduces infant anxiety, and lastly reduces maternal breast-cancer risk. There is a more beneficial nutrigenomic and epigenetic effect (helpful expression of DNA) when an infant is breastfed vs. formula fed. Formula has its place when breast milk can't be provided, or a mother is a heroin addict, but it should not be promoted above and beyond an available natural solution.

Thank you for letting me share my perspectives! I encourage everyone to critically analyze the data, and to avoid being unduly influenced by the opinions of corporations or lobby groups that are biased by greed and power. We can fix our broken system, but we must vote smart and speak out to legislators to seek the change that's needed. Let's go primal now!

The Coming Re-emergence of Ancient Medicine and Spirituality

It may be time to consider a new therapeutic gestalt, thus giving greater credence to ancient healing modalities. For those simply seeking a spiritual transformation, the use of psychoactive plants under the guidance of a qualified shaman may offer a deeper root or connectedness to the world around you. Further, in many academic and medical circles psychoactive plants are considered entheogens—the Greek word *entheogen* means "awakening or generating the divine within." Certain plant entheogens are known to contain psychoactive substances that may produce a profound spiritual experience, deepening your connection with self, the universe, oneness, and God. This contrasts with tripping out via recreational use of drugs or plants.

Entheogens are typically held in sacred space by shamans, curanderos, or healers, who, generally speaking, help to set an intention and should not have a malevolent agenda.

In sacred spaces, with intention and mindfulness, mystical experiences can occur. Examples might be prayer, meditation, breathwork, visits to sacred sites, work with psychoactive plants, and many more. A mystical experience oftentimes reveals your inner god, spirit, and interconnections to the cosmos. Benevolent deities, saints, and spirit entities may offer healings, creative insights, and downloads.

According to Albert Einstein, "The most important and profound emotion that we can experience is the sensation of the mystical. It is the source of all true science . . . To know that what is impenetrable to us really exists, manifesting itself as the highest wisdom and the most radiant beauty."[234]

One must be willing to let go and allow the psychoactive plant and curandero to assist in your mystical healing—and spirit travel into what is, in our conscious states, typically an impenetrable portal. To give you a feel for what I am describing, I've detailed one of my Peruvian ayahuasca ceremonies below.

My Personal Experience with Ayahuasca

Many years ago I took this personal challenge and traveled to Peru, not to simply see the famed and mysterious Machu Picchu, but more importantly to make a quantum leap in my spiritual growth. I'd been feeling a disconnect from my deeper self, nature, God, and the cosmos after being confined in fluorescent-lit rooms, seeing patients day to day. I wasn't seeking a reboot from the end of a relationship, as Elizabeth Gilbert dialogues in *Eat, Pray, Love*, but was seeking a nourishing infusion of primal spiritual connection to the earth and stars.

After the rigorous hike of the Inca Trail, followed by touring and connecting with the energies of Machu Picchu, I decided I needed to tap into dimensions beyond our 3-D world with the help of a Shipibo shaman, who was offering ayahuasca ceremonies near Pisac. Traditionally, he would perform these in the rainforest, but had brought his vine to another powerful region of Peru, known as the Sacred Valley. According to the Ayahuasca Legal Defense Fund, ceremonial use of ayahuasca is legal in Peru, supported by their government and the medical and spiritual community as being a therapeutic medicine.

Prior to participating, I had to maintain a strict diet for a few days, drinking only mineral water the last twenty-four hours. The shaman also assisted me in making *despacho*, or offerings, to the Inca gods the afternoon before the ceremony. On this auspicious evening almost ten years ago, I found myself in a circular ceremony room in the Sacred Valley of Peru. A fire burned in the center of the room and I found myself not in a large circle of twenty, as often happens, but by myself—attended by one Shipibo shaman and a female apprentice. Personalized attention for sure! The Shipibo's lineage, knowledge, medicine, and relationship with this plant made it the closest thing to being in the rainforest. His face was weathered, and I estimated him to be in his seventies. His eyes, and energy field emanated wisdom and interdimensional connectedness.

Despite feeling comfortable with his presence and grateful for the gift of individualized care, being alone without other Westerners had me feeling a bit uneasy. The shamans had made a sacred brew from the ayahuasca vine by boiling it, then combining it with a plant called *chacruna*, which synergistically creates this medicine. What's mind-boggling is the Amazon rainforest is estimated to have more than 80,000 plant species.[235] How the shamans isolated these two plants and figured out how to make this sacred brew is a mystery that's frequently debated amongst anthropologists.

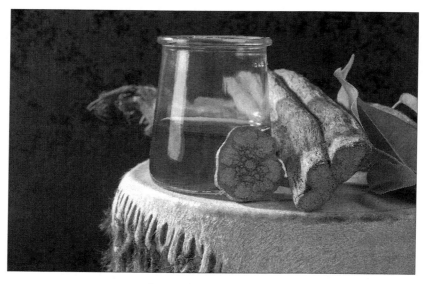

Ayahuasca brew (Shutterstock)

At sunset, with the fire stoked in the center of the circular ceremonial room warming the cool room, I could hear the valley breeze blowing down from the Andes Mountains around us, rustling the thatched roof above. I could hear a donkey hee-hawing in a nearby pasture. Wrapped in beautiful, bright colored, geometrically patterned, lama-wool Peruvian blankets, I sat in fear on a meditation pillow. Thoughts began to run through my head:

How crazy for me to do this! I could die or maybe flip out on this journey. This could change me forever. I centered myself and began a slow-breathing meditation to relax. I was told I had to trust in "Grandmother," the medicine, and to speak my intention, but also allow her to do the needed work. It was similar to running off a cliff to paraglide. For a successful flight, you have to trust, let go, and flow with the whole process.

As the fire danced in front of my eyes, and the smoke snaked to the opening in the thatched roof, flowing to the stars on this clear crisp night, the elder shaman began singing icaros to the medicine. The icaros are songs created by the Quechua-speaking people of the Amazon to activate the maroon-colored medicine in circle. Soon he offered me a few ounces. Swallowing quickly, I chased the bittersweet taste down with water and then waited in silence as more icaros were chanted to activate the medicine. First, the sound calmed the nausea from the medicine. For almost an hour I sat listening and staring at the dancing flames, wondering if anything was going to happen. Suddenly, over a period of minutes, I started seeing geometry—predominately hexagons— then three-dimensional shapes morphing into tetrahedrons and other complex forms.

The geometry came alive, with gold light intermixed with iridescent, fluorescent-like colors of unbelievable beauty. At times multidimensional-seeming, it took me on a fractal trail that seemed to go to infinity. I felt a deep oneness with the universe. Miniscule, segmented, snake-like forms appeared and traveled though my body, as if scanning my meridian lines. At one point, I could visualize them scanning through the double helix of my DNA—mending, then removing unwanted DNA fragments.

I journeyed into the other dimensions for a few hours—boosted even more deeply with an extra dose—visualizing things that would take another book to describe. A few times, the periodic intense waves of nausea almost made me throw up, but calmed by the icaros, I held on a little longer. With my eyes closed, I noticed how the energy of the song intensified the geometry. When he stopped, the visual intensity of colors and geometry would drop off by at least one-third. Never had I imagined that sound would so profoundly increase the visual complexity and color saturation. This enhancement occurred with perfect synchrony to his chanting.

As the medicine and icaros continued their healing, I came to a distinct point where I knew it was time to clear out and release what my physical, mental, and spiritual body no longer needed. Intense nausea hit me and I quickly grabbed the bucket beside me to purge. I thought I would see the medicine coming up. But to my amazement, a black hole-like vortex appeared in the middle of the bucket, funneling this unwanted matter into another dimension. Perhaps a cosmic dumpster! I could see it circling down the vortex just as water spirals down and out of a funnel, followed by the bucket then reappearing.

After this journey, I became convinced that plants, especially ayahuasca, can favorably affect our DNA. In my case, in a cleansing of negative energies. Seeing the enhancement and increased complexity of geometry and color through music and chanting, I realized how—as we process these higher levels of light and geometry—sound can further stimulate our brain and likely our DNA. The out-of-body visualization of my energy field confirmed my belief in the Chinese acupuncture meridian system and the Ayurvedic chakra-based system.

Additional work with this sacred plant in Peru has produced similar experiences and greater insights. Every one of them unique with varied intensities and insights coming in. About a year later I picked up Jeremy Narby's *The Cosmic Serpent: DNA and the Origins of Knowledge* (1998). As an anthropologist, deep in the jungle with Amazonian Shipibo shamans, Narby studied the medicinal benefits of ayahuasca.

To my surprise Narby—eloquently and with great depth—describes the same fluorescent snakes I'd seen! He saw them as DNA-like—insightfully making the comparison: "DNA is the snake-shaped master of transformation that lives in water and is both extremely long and small, single and double. Just like the cosmic serpent . . . DNA is compared not only to two entwined serpents, but also precisely, to a rope, a vine, a ladder or a stairway."[236] As I looked at Jeremy's experience beside mine, the only difference was that the minute snakes were scanning and repairing my helical DNA rather than actually *being* DNA.

In *The Way of the Shaman: a Guide to Power and Healing* (1980), Michael Harner describes how the majority of shamans he interviewed had seen, like him, colorful serpents. Harner documents the presence of the cosmic serpent—including Ronin, the Amazonian two-headed anaconda; Quetzalcoatl, the Aztec feathered serpent; the Rainbow Snake of the Australian aborigines; the cosmic serpent of ancient Egyptians; the thousand-headed serpent god Sesha of the Hindus; and others. This intrigued me, as I'd been having dreams about Quetzalcoatl.

As mentioned in Chapter 5 ("Sound: Creator and Healer"), to the Maya, the plumed serpent Kukulkan is revered at the step pyramid (El Castillo) in Chichen Itza, where annually during the fall and spring equinox, watched by thousands, the shadow of the serpent appears on the side of the temple.

Prior to reading Narby, I had a meditative insight to reconnect the energies of the eagle and the condor by placing Lemurian crystals at sacred sites—Machu Picchu, Peru; then Palenque, Mexico; Chaco Canyon; Mount Shasta; Rapa Nui (Easter Island), and many others. Deep in meditation, I occasionally see the plumed serpent flying over these sacred sites and feel that the spirit of Kukulkan is perhaps helping to reconnect them along sacred ley lines. Now this grid of crystals has extended to over fifty sacred locations. You can see the current Google map of my grid through the link on my spiritual genomics website.[237]

Ayahuasca Brewing and Properties

Ayahuasca tea is brewed by breaking up and boiling the sacred vine (Banisiteriopsis caapi) and typically adding leaves from the chacruna shrub (Psychotria viridis) that contains DMT (dimethyltryptamine). DMT, an entheogen, has a stimulating effect on the pineal gland, the deep interior organ in the brain often identified with the Third Eye in the Hindu chakra system. The Greek word *entheogen* (as mentioned, it means "generating the divine within") includes all the molecules discussed in this chapter. Some, like MDMA, are primarily empathogens, enhancing connectedness, heart openness, and compassion.

Holistic health coach Joshua Eagle, author of *Mind Nutrition: Timeless Secrets to Enhance Your Brain Daily*, connects ayahuasca to the timely topic of methylation. He says, "One of the main modes in which Ayahuasca works to clean out the pineal gland and brain is through the act of methylation. . . . Methyl-donors in our body, which work to identify toxins and route them out for elimination, can become depleted when one's body encounters too much toxicity for the liver to handle. It is in these circumstances where plants containing an abundance of methyl-donors are particularly helpful." Where can one get these methyl-donors? Eagle explains:

> The top three foods containing methyl-donors in order are: 1) Ayahuasca, 2) Beets and 3) Goji Berries.
>
> The specific methylating compound in Ayahuasca which works to jump-start this detoxification process is frequently referred to as DMT or di-methyl-tryptamine. The DMT molecule—which is found present in every single living animal and plant—only becomes bioavailable when it is combined with an MAO-inhibitor plant that prevents it from being too rapidly metabolized by the body. In the case of Ayahuasca, the Chakruna leaf is the DMT containing plant and the Ayahuasca contains the MAO-inhibiting properties which allows for the DMT to become bioavailable."[238]

One of the most common conditions I address with natural remedies in my practice is methylation disorders. Depending on the type of involvement/impairment of the methylene tetrahydrofolate reductase (MTHFR) enzyme, individuals may have an increase in depression, anxiety, autism, blood clots, cancer, neural tube defects, Crohn's disease, etc.[239] Identifying and addressing this genetic defect with a simple, bioactive folate supplement, such as L-methylfolate, with cofactors at the appropriate dose—

combined with other nutritional support—can oftentimes resolve their condition. In my opinion, those suffering from MTHFR gene involvement with depression may benefit from methylation-support plant medications in addition to methylfolate. Of course, prior to proceeding, discuss this with your physician and other therapists involved. For a great review of MTHFR gene-mutation types and other genes implicated in methylation and detoxification, I recommend visiting the website of Ben Lynch, ND (http://mthfr.net), and reading his new book, *Dirty Genes.*

DMT

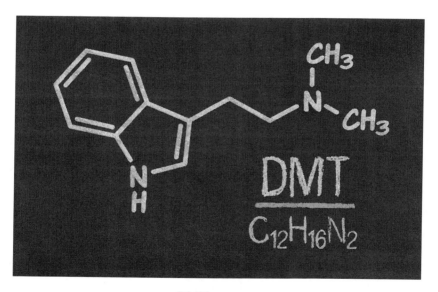

DMT structure

DMT, or N, N-Dimethyltryptamine, a tryptamine molecule, is found (and can be isolated) in many species of plants and animals. In sacred circles it's commonly combined with the Amazonian ayahuasca brew, as mentioned, but has also been isolated from the glands of the Sonoran Desert toad or chemically synthesized for mystical experiences.

DMT likely possesses the most potent spiritual and ego-dissolving properties of all molecules discussed. Pure forms that are smoked or that have been given by IV in research are broken down quickly by MAO (Monoamine oxidase) enzymes, lasting typically only fifteen minutes. Thousands of years ago the Amazonian Shipibo tribe enigmatically figured out how to prolong the duration of plant-based DMT without the help of a modern lab! They continue to do this today by combining the MAO properties of the Banisteriopsis caapi vine, which prevent the breakdown of DMT, with the DMT-rich Psychotric Viridis (chacruna plant), creating ayahuasca that has hours instead of minutes of duration.

Whether seeking a long journey with the Amazonian brew or doing a short DMT journey, both send individuals deeper into the cosmos. Ayahuasca gives a more gradual spiral into the cosmic realms, whereas pure DMT rockets one into these realms with what many would describe as the white light of a near-death experience. Both speeds have been observed to connect people intimately with oneness. Most who work with this pure form of DMT smoke it ceremonially and typically experience a brief journey, unless a "second pipe" is utilized.

Rick Strassman, clinical associate professor of psychiatry at the University of New Mexico, was curious whether during mystical states and psychedelic experiences the pineal gland itself produces DMT. He hypothesized that the pineal has *light* sensitivity and is responsible for the production and release of DMT, an entheogen that, he believes, could be excreted in large quantities at the moments of birth and death.

Beginning in 1990, for five years Dr. Strassman administered approximately four hundred intravenous doses to sixty human volunteers in a federal-government-funded project at the General Clinical Research Center of the University of New Mexico Hospital. In *DMT: The Spirit Molecule: A Doctor's Revolutionary Research into the Biology of Near-Death and Mystical Experiences*, he says, "This molecule provides our consciousness access to the most amazing and unexpected visions, thoughts, and feelings. It throws open the door to worlds beyond our imagination."[240]

Alexander and Ann Shulgin discuss DMT's ubiquitous presence in nature in their book *TIHKAL: The Continuation.* (THIKAL stands for "Tryptamines I Have Known and Loved.") DMT is found, they wrote, "in this flower here, in that tree over there, and in yonder animal. It is, most simply everywhere you choose to look."[241] According to Dr. Strassman, "Equally important is that DMT occurs in our bodies. It may be upon endogenous DMT wings that we experience other life-changing states of mind associated with birth, death, and near death, entity or alien contact experiences, and mystical/spiritual consciousness."[242] He also noted: "DMT is the simplest of the tryptamine psychedelics . . . and is rather small. DMT is closely related to serotonin, the neurotransmitter that psychedelics affect so widely."[243] Beyond our brain and nervous system, receptors for serotonin can be found in our GI tract, vessels, skin, and glands.

The first in twenty years to legally do research in the U.S. that involved giving participants psychedelics, Strassman fought hard to get to that point. Funding was not easy to come by. His work is widely credited with leading the way to a revival of scientific study of the "spirit molecule" and other entheogens.

302

In the spring of 2016 at the Hotel Boulderado I attended a lecture by Dr. Strassman, where he updated passionate psychedelic attendees on the latest findings in DMT research and its impact on human consciousness. He stated that DMT is mainly produced in the lungs, and that recent research has found the enzymes and precursors for it in the lungs. Answering many questions from the audience, he stated that he's unsure if fluoride in our water has an adverse effect on our pineal and DMT release; he agreed with an attendee that DMT can change our minds in a way that makes us want to protect this molecule. I feel our relationship with DMT, whether enhanced by breathwork or other modality, brings us closer to God, and thus to our community and the environment. By protecting and showing others how to commune with the spirit molecule we are evolving ourselves further along a path of altruism and love.

According to his research, "The brain is where DMT exerts its most interesting effects. Although the brain denies access to most drugs and chemicals, it takes a particular and remarkable fancy to DMT. It is not stretching the truth to suggest that the brain 'hungers' for it.'"[244]

How do DMT and psychedelic plants act on serotonin in our brain and nervous system, compared to antidepressants? The most common antidepressants are SSRIs. SSRIs (selective serotonin reuptake inhibitors)—such as Prozac, Paxil, Zoloft—block the reuptake of the serotonin neurotransmitter at the presynaptic cell, thereby resulting in more serotonin being available to be received at the postsynaptic receptor.

Just think of me as a lousy tennis player who has a ball thrower inundating me with hundreds of tennis balls, and I can only get a few of them back over the net. SSRIs act like a big net, keeping the balls in my court, surrounding me (the postsynaptic cell) with more serotonin to improve my mood. But with psychedelic plants, LSD, and DMT, I don't need a net to keep more serotonin in my court, because they act like additional serotonin tennis balls that have a different color (structure) and bind to slightly different serotonin receptors. If LSD and other "balls" in this category were coming at me, they'd stick to me like Velcro and interact more robustly with my body. They'd bind to various serotonin receptors on the postsynaptic membrane, particularly the 5-HT2A receptor.

At lower doses this more direct serotonin agonist interaction with these receptors promotes empathy and enhanced mood. At higher doses a mystical and psychedelic state is often experienced. This may include seeing vivid colors and geometry, for example.

The psilocybin mushroom has more mixed serotonin agonist activity. The activity of LSD and these Tryptan-like psychoactive plants eventually wears off, as an enzyme called MAO (Monoamine oxidase) breaks it down. In fact, ayahuasca works by blocking the breakdown of DMT plants included in the brew, thus allowing for a more sustained, four-hour journey.

Huachuma (San Pedro Cactus)

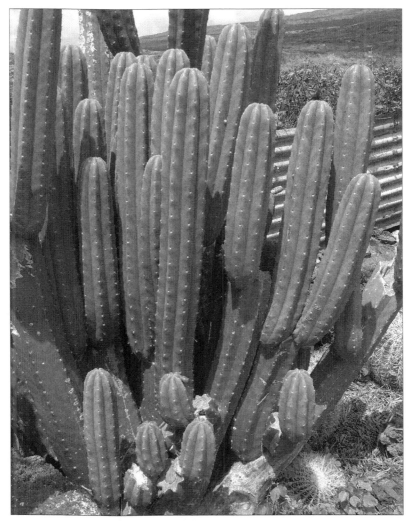

Huachuma cactus. Photo by Forest & Kim Starr, Wikimedia Commons.

In the high Andes of Peru and Ecuador, historically, for three thousand years, the cactus Huachuma (San Pedro) was used to shamanically connect humans to Mother Earth and the upper world. This tea is typically consumed in a daytime ceremony rather than nighttime, unlike ayahuasca.

The earliest archaeological evidence discovered is a stone carving of a Huachumero found at the Jaguar Temple of Chavín de Huantar in northern Peru. Textiles from the same region and period of history depict the cactus with jaguars and hummingbirds, two of its guardian spirits, and with spiral symbols, representing its ability to produce a visionary experience.

Huachuma ceremonies where the plant is consumed as a tea are still held today in parts of the world. These ceremonies may cure illness of a spiritual, emotional, mental, or physical nature. They may illuminate the future through prophetic and divinatory qualities of the plant, assist one to overcome sorcery or saladera, to ensure success in one's ventures, to rekindle love and enthusiasm for life and to experience the world as divine. The San Pedro cactus brings in the masculine energy of the Heavens (from above), contrasting it to Ayahuasca which brings in the feminine energy of Mother Earth (from below).

One Andean shaman describes some of the effects of the plant: "First, a dreamy state . . . then great visions, a clearing of all the faculties . . . and then detachment, a type of visual force inclusive of the sixth sense, the telepathic state of transmitting oneself across time and matter, like a removal of thoughts to a distant dimension."[245]

Working with it personally in Peru many years ago and where it is legal, I've experienced much of what he describes as well as the most loving connection to nature I've ever experienced. On the trails I found myself pausing to hug trees, feeling a deep grounding as I put my arms around them or placed my forehead lightly against the bark of the trunk. Just to touch any tree, plant, or rock while on this medicine precipitates an interchange of loving energy to Mother Earth. With your qi, prana, or life force more open, you connect with nature more flowingly than in an ordinary state of consciousness. I even witnessed a faint glow or aura around the trees and plants, and was mesmerized by the finer details in leaves—their fractal geometry. While this can be experienced with psilocybin and others, I found huachuma gave me a quantum leap. The colors in flowers became more vivid and glowing, and I perceived the leaves taking in the photons of energy from the sun.

Oftentimes as I connected to the plants and earth during a twelve-hour-plus journey, I've felt an intensified kundalini flow, which I had to ground out by lying on the ground, or—to mitigate the intense streaming of energy from my hands and body—drop into yoga poses such as Downward-facing Dog.

With my hands and feet electrified, this allowed for an open flow to ground out the intense energy into Gaia. As with other psychoactive plants, the ego dissolves, replaced by a sense of oneness with Planet Earth and the infinite universe. When nightfall came, I experienced geometry as complex and colorful as with ayahuasca. In summary, the benefits include improving the flow from root to crown chakra, bridging a deep connection between Mother Earth and, simultaneously, the geometry and energies from the upper world in a more subtle way than with ayahuasca. As with the other plants, one may become detached from ego, traveling to beyond-3-D dimensions, receiving insights and deep healing. Despite the intensity of a huachuma journey, one is less likely to purge than in an ayahuasca ceremony. Its bitterness can produce some nausea.

Psilocybin

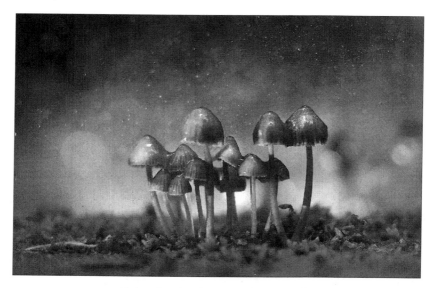

Psilocybin mushroom (Shutterstock)

For at least two thousand years psilocybin has been used by Native American cultures—Aztec, Maya. Over two hundred species of mushrooms on our planet contain this psychedelic compound.[246] Fungi in general, have been present on our planet for over 600 million years and have played an extremely important role in the evolution of plants and animals.

New research from the University of Valladoid in Spain, published in the *Daily Mail* June 27, 2018, was headlined: NO WON-

DER THEY CALLED IT THE STONE AGE—ANCIENT HUMANS WERE TAKING DRUGS—INCLUDING MAGIC MUSHROOMS AND OPIUM—UP TO 10,600 YEARS AGO. The research, revealed in *Time and Mind*, reported on the ancient use of psychedelics in different parts of the world:

> Early humans also used hallucinogenic plants, according to Professor Guerra-Doce.
>
> There is evidence dating back to between 8,600 BC and 5,600 BC that ancient inhabitants of caves in Peru's Callejon de Huaylas Valley were using Echinopsis pachanoi—a cactus that contains the psychedelic substance mescaline.
>
> Archaeologists have found traces of the cactus and pollen in the Guitarrero cave in the area.
>
> Researchers have also found reddish stains on 13,000-year-old human teeth found in a burial pit in Duyong Cave on Palawan Island in the southern Philippines, which are thought to be caused by chewing the leaves of the betel plant. . . .
>
> Magic mushrooms have also been commonly used throughout history, according to Professor Guerra-Doce.
>
> Mushroom shaped carvings into rocky outcrops dating from the Neolithic and Bronze Age in northwest Piedmont in the Italian Alps, have been interpreted as signs that psychotropic mushrooms were used in rituals.

The use of hallucinogenic mushrooms has also been documented by small sculptures that resemble mushrooms which have been found at numerous sites dating back to between 500 BC and 900 AD in Guatemala, Mexico, Honduras and El Salvador.

Given its prolific presence on all continents except Antarctica for thousands of years, one can guess that psilocybin has been the most globally used psychoactive organism.

Francis Crick, co-discoverer of DNA, asked, sometime back, whether an advanced civilization planted primitive spores of life on a rocket, thus seeding our planet with DNA from outside our atmosphere. Carefully scientific, he said, along with British chemist Leslie Orgel, at a conference on Communication with Extraterrestrial Intelligence organized by American astronomer, astrophysicist, astrobiologist Carl Sagan in 1971 in Soviet Armenia, the theory of direct panspermia—though not certain—was "plausible."[247] He did not mention psilocybin.

Terence McKenna, ethnobotanist, mystic, psychonaut, and author of *Food of the Gods: The Search for the Original Tree of Knowledge A Radical History of Plants, Drugs, and Human Evolution*, researched "the powerful potential to replace abuse of illegal drugs with a shamanic understanding, insistence on community, reverence for nature, and increased self-awareness." He advocated for the use of psychedelic plants responsibly. Panspermia is the theory that microorganisms and other forms of life may have arrived by asteroid or meteorite from within or outside our galaxy. Wikipedia notes:

> In a more radical version of biophysicist Francis Crick's hypothesis of directed panspermia, McK-

enna speculated on the idea that psilocybin mushrooms may be a species of high intelligence, which may have arrived on this planet as spores migrating through space and which are attempting to establish a symbiotic relationship with human beings. He postulated that "intelligence, not life, but intelligence may have come here [to Earth] in this spore-bearing life form." He said, "I think that theory will probably be vindicated. I think in a hundred years if people do biology they will think it quite silly that people once thought that spores could not be blown from one star system to another by cosmic radiation pressure."

Did psilocybin help mankind and other animals evolve over millions of years, as has been hypothesized? According to McKenna, in his "stoned ape theory," not only humans but also other animal species likely gained evolutionary benefits from it. Below is a colorful summary:

McKenna posited that psilocybin caused the primitive brain's information-processing capabilities to rapidly reorganize, which in turn kick-started the rapid evolution of cognition that led to the early art, language, and technology written in Homo sapiens' archeological record. As early humans, he said, we "ate our way to higher consciousness" by consuming these mushrooms, which, he hypothesized, grew out of animal manure. Psilocybin, he said, brought us "out of the animal mind and into the world of articulated speech and imagination."

As human cultural evolution led to the domestication of wild cattle, humans began to spend a lot more time around cattle dung, McKenna explained. And, because psilocybin mushrooms commonly grow in cow droppings, "the human-mushroom interspecies codependency was enhanced and deepened. It was at this time that religious ritual, calendar making, and natural magic came into their own."[248]

At the Psychedelic Science conference in 2017, Dr. Paul Stamets, world famous mycologist, author, and expert on psilocybin, revived the more or less defunct theory because of a new discovery: "What is really important for you to understand is that there was a sudden doubling of the human brain 200,000 years ago. From an evolutionary point of view, that's an extraordinary expansion. And there is no explanation for this sudden increase in the human brain."[249]

Oxford neurobiologist Colin Blakemore likewise asked, in a recent lecture, why is it our brain had a gradual increase in size, starting three million years ago? Then, abruptly, there was a remarkable increase "of about 30% or so." He hypothesizes a different instigator than psilocybin.[250]

My opinion is that we co-evolved with fungi and everything around us. A combination of better hunting and cultivation/sourcing enhanced our intake of healthy protein and plants (nutrigenomic effect). Further stimuli for cortical brain growth included environmental stressors (epigenetic effect), requiring greater problem-solving skills, language, and social, and spiritual growth. To integrate and further catalyze this growth while quenching our thirst for understanding consciousness, early and contemporary humans have used "mind expanding" fungi and plants as allies to evolve spiritually and improve creativity. These provide for greater psychological stability and improved problem-solving. Both are critical to our survival.

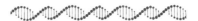

While visiting Vietnam years ago with a spiritual group of twenty, I decided to try the psilocybin mushroom. It's legal there and was offered to us by a shaman. Afterwards, hiking in the rainforest, I was able to see things with improved acuity. This enhancement to our visual cortex is similar to what one experiences with an improved prescription for glasses or contacts, but with better color and improved detection of movement. I could see how hunters would benefit.

As an avid amateur photographer, I've loved the high-dynamic-range (i.e., more vivid color depth) images possible with newer high-end cameras. I hypothesize that psilocybin provides humans with this enhancement by upscaling our brain's capacity to process more visual data, while at the same time improving our processing speed. It's also similar to what one gets by upgrading the processor, graphic card, and monitor on a dated computer. Similar to the San Pedro cactus in Peru, this mushroom made me want to feel nature and commune with it—sliding off my shoes and walking barefoot on the ground, letting the energy flow through my feet and up my spine. There was a deeper, more intimate flow of appreciation to the trees and plants around me in that Vietnam forest, sometimes prompting me to place my forehead on a tree and flow into its roots below and canopy above.

The fractal growth of the roots and branches, I felt more energetically. Birds and other animals I encountered didn't spook and run, but stared at me deeply. Rather than being seen as a predator, I was seen as one with them.

As I felt a more intimate relationship to nature I could see how it would make an individual or culture more nurturing and protective of the fragile environment. Of course, perhaps the mushroom has a self-preserving interest by promoting these effects on our brains for their own habitat protection. Just as flowers provide nectar for bees to pollinate and proliferate their species

With psilocybin, it's very possible to go into that egoless state of oneness.

Unfortunately, the transformative psilocybin mushroom species is currently categorized as a Schedule 1 drug in the U.S., thus illegal. Based on very promising research demonstrating its antidepressant and spiritual benefits, Denver now has a ballot initiative to be voted on in May 2019 to make psilocybin the lowest law-enforcement priority—in effect, decriminalized. I've been supportive of the MAPS group and others to help make this a reality, sooner rather than later.

To return now to the Marsh Chapel experiment, or "Miracle of Marsh Chapel," which took place in 1962 at Harvard University. In that study, with Timothy Leary and Richard Alpert as advisors, Walter Pahnke's tests showed that during a Good Friday service a genuine religious experience was facilitated when a hallucinogenic plant was administered just beforehand. Ten control-group participants from Andover-Newton Theological Seminary took active niacin—which would produce tingling. Only one had a mystical or religious experience, while eight or nine of the ten who took thirty milligrams of psilocybin did. The feelings they experienced included sacredness, ineffability, and a sense of oneness with the divine. An interesting outcome is that nine of the ten divinity students who took psilocybin became ordained ministers, whereas the ten in the placebo group did not complete the path of ordination.[251] Fast forward forty years. A groundbreaking study picked up where Pahnke left off.

In 2002, Roland Griffiths, a behavioral scientist, undertook an in-depth look at psilocybin's effect on consciousness. Griffiths had started his career in behavioral medicine but in an unlikely detour became interested in Siddha Yoga in 1994, which led him to meditate and study Eastern traditions. This eventually induced a sense of malaise in his work. He even considered changing jobs. And then came a chance to study psilocybin.

His results were published in *Psychopharmacology* (2006), as "Psilocybin Can Occasion Mystical-Type Experiences Having Substantial and Sustained Personal Meaning and Spiritual Significance." And in 2008: "Mystical-Type Experiences Occasioned by Psilocybin Mediate the Attribution of Personal Meaning and Spiritual Significance 14 Months Later." The work was hailed as "the first rigorously designed, double-blind, placebo-controlled clinical study in more than four decades—if not ever—to examine the psychological effects of a psychedelic."[252]

Results indicated that psilocybin can create substantial personal meaning and significance, sustained even fourteen months out. A very high percentage of participants found the experience amongst the top five most meaningful in their life.[253]

Again, in a study published in 2016, "Psilocybin Produces Substantial and Sustained Decreases in Depression and Anxiety in Patients with Life-threatening Cancer: A Randomized Double-Blind Trial," Griffiths was lead researcher. In this Johns Hopkins experiment, fifty-one cancer patients with a life-threatening diagnosis and symptoms of depression and anxiety were administered psilocybin in a randomized, controlled trial. Enhancements in well-being, life satisfaction, relationships, spirituality, and mystical experiences were noted.[254]

Michael Pollan, professor of journalism at Berkeley, is the author of seven *New York Times* best sellers. He discusses the history, personal journeys, and responsible use of LSD, psilocybin, and DMT in his new book, *How to Change Your Mind: What the New Science of Psychedelics Teaches Us about Consciousness, Dying, Addiction, Depression, and Transcendence* (2018). Opening the topic to his more mainstream audience, he describes the resurgent interest in these psychedelic compounds in ongoing clinical trials.

Pollan has this to say about one of his journeys: "Like one of those flimsy wooden houses erected on Bikini Atoll to be blown up in the nuclear tests, 'I' was no more, blasted to a confetti cloud."[255] The ego dies, but you still perceive a consciousness, he writes. With psilocybin, he says, the "Default Mode Network," which includes brain structures such as the prefrontal cortex and posterior cingulate cortex, are taken offline—dissolving the ego, enhancing creativity, and making the experiencer let go of time. As he explained, the brain scans of individuals on a psilocybin journey look very similar to the brain of an experienced meditator going deep. Paul Expert, a neurobiologist complexity researcher at the Imperial College of London, and his team imaged the brains of fifteen individuals via fMRI scans on and off psilo-cybin. The results were fascinating![256]

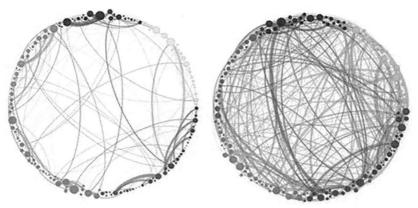

Communication between brain networks in people given psilocybin
(right) or a nonpsychedelic compound (left). Petri et al.
Proceedings of the Royal Society Interface.

They found that the brain still maintains organizational features while taking psilocybin, while at the same time demonstrating enhanced activity in nonlinear process regions of the brain, promoting "outside of the box" thinking.

A recent documentary, *A New Understanding: The Science of Psilocybin*, investigates its medical effect. The film quotes David Nutt, a professor of neuropsychopharmacology in the division of brain sciences at Imperial College London: "Psilocybin does in 30 seconds what antidepressants take three to four weeks to do." The report of the film in *Business Insider* goes on: "Researchers have found that a single dose of psilocybin accompanied by therapy can have a transformational effect on mental health—like a 'surgical intervention'—able to treat even cases of depression and anxiety that resist standard treatment."

Explaining further, David Nichols, president and co-founder of the Heffter Research Institute, adds: "In order to cause these effects, these drugs activate serotonin 2a receptors." He says: "But something about this experience—the brain activation, illusions, and hallucinations—seems to do something more profound that's harder to understand. It's able to reliably cause what researchers call a 'mystical experience.' That experience is strongly linked with lasting effects."[257]

In conversation with Michael Pollan, Paul Stamets said, "Plants and mushrooms have intelligence, and they want us to take care of the environment, and so they communicate that to us in a way we can understand . . . we just need to be better listeners."[258]

In my opinion, future legalization of psilocybin offers the greatest potential benefit to society due to its therapeutic capacity, low side-effect profile, nonaddictive properties, affordability, and most importantly its capacity to reconnect us to ourselves, nature, and one another.

Peyote (Lophophora Williamsii)

Peyote is a well-known, small, spineless cactus native to Mexico and southwestern Texas, whose medicinal and spiritual use dates back over fifty-five hundred years there, as confirmed by researchers when they found peyote buttons at Shumla Cave No. 5 on the Rio Grande in Texas.[259]

Like the Peruvian San Pedro cactus, it contains psychoactive mescaline. The Native American Nahuatl name, *peyotl*, translates to "Divine Messenger."[260] During ceremonial use this psychoactive plant produces rich visions or auditory effects and may help with pain, fever, skin conditions, rheumatism, colds, and diabetes.[261]

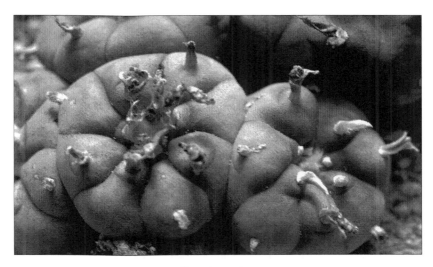

Peyote cactus

Firsthand accounts of indigenous use of peyote go back to Friar Bernadino de] Sahagun Sahagún (1499–1590)—not published till centuries later. He spent much of his adulthood in Mexico among the Chichimeca and wrote: "There is another herb like tunas [Opuntia spp.] of the earth. It is called Peiotl. It is white. It is found in the north country. Those who eat or drink it see visions either frightful or laughable. This intoxication lasts two or three days and then ceases. It is a common food of the Chichimeca, for it sustains them and gives them courage to fight and not feel fear nor hunger nor thirst. And they say that it protects them from all danger."[262]

Because it was taken to be holy medicine, "the underlying belief in the supernatural origin of visions is important among factors contributing to the diffusion of peyote and, in a general way, defines the area of its probable spread."

The following data and excerpts are from "The Appeal of Peyote (Lophophora Williamsii) as a Medicine," published in the *American Anthropologist* by Richard Evans Schultes, Harvard educator and American biologist, the "father of modern ethnobotany.[263] Schultes looked at books in part written in the sixteenth century, including one by Spanish king Philip II's personal physician, Francisco Hernández de Toledo.

In 1570, under orders to do the earliest scientific study of the New World medicinal plants and animals, Hernández sailed there from Europe. Besides collecting three thousand species, he did interviews with indigenous people and performed medical studies.[264]

> The medico-religious peyote cult was already estab-
> lished in Mexico when the Spaniards arrived. The
> earliest record of the use of *Lophophora Williamsii*
> is that of [friar Bernadino de] Sahagun who wrote
> that the Chichimeca [eight indigenous nations] ate
> the root, peiotl, which induced amusing or terrifying
> visions and stimulated them in battle. . . .
>
> Hernández, describing the plant as *Peyotl zacate-*
> *censis,* emphasized the fact that it was used in
> prophesying and in the treatment of pains. He did
> not mention peyote visions.
>
> Likewise, [Father José] Ortego, who described the
> Cora ceremony, made no mention of visions. Fur-
> thermore, [Franciscan theologian José] Arlegui did
> not report visual hallucinations, but stated emphati-
> cally that peyote was administered as a panacea and
> as an aid in prophesying.

Thus, from a survey of early Mexican accounts of the use of peyote, the importance of the plant as a medicine seems to overtop the importance of peyote visions.[265]

Continuing on into today, peyote is widely used in a ceremonial and religious context in the U.S. and Mexico among its adherents:

> That the therapeutic appeal of *Lophophora WIliarn-sii* is still strong in Mexico is shown by recent writers. Lumholtz wrote that the Tarahumare, Huichol, and Tepehuane apply peyote externally for rheumatism, wounds, burns, snakebites, and skin diseases. Furthermore, he stated that "it is an absolute cure against the painful stings of scorpions, and, as such, deserves to be widely known." Bennett and Zingg have found that the Tarahumare apply crushed peyote externally as an ointment. In this tribe "hicouri (peyote) dances are more frequent during times of sickness." Peyote has been widely used in Mexico as a cure for arrow wounds; the dried, powdered root being packed into the wound until healing occurs.
>
> In Mexico, as in the United States, the therapeutic use of *Lophophora Williamsii* grades into the superstitious and pseudotherapeutic. To its use is attributed health and longevity; rubbed on the knees, it is believed to give strength in walking; in curing disease, it is said to fortify the body against future ills and to purify the soul.

The creative stimulation is best represented through the art of the Huichol natives of central-western Mexico, who have been using peyote for over fifteen thousand years. Their colorful, beaded animals on wood can be found in many galleries carrying Mexicana art. Jaguar heads, beaded eggs, yarn paintings, ceremonial bowls, and figurines are also noteworthy.

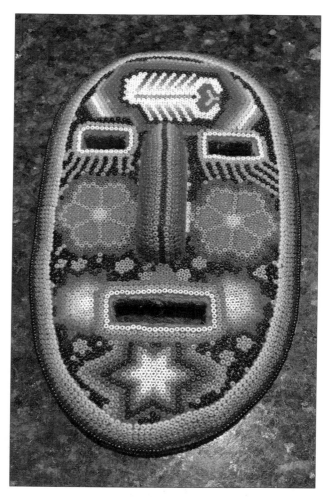

Huichol peyote mask. Photo by the
author of a mask he purchased.

322

"The primary event in Huichol religious practice is the peyote hunt, an annual pilgrimage that acts out a desire to return to the source of all life and heal oneself. For the hunt, Huichol travel 300 miles to their paradise, Wirikuta." There they hunt for their yearly supply of peyote.[266] Peyote is a visionary sacrament for them, as well as for many other Native American cultures.

To Americans, peyote might be best known through the writings of anthropologist Carlos Castaneda, such as *The Teachings of Don Juan*, which have sold 28 million copies. His teacher was a Yaqui "Man of Knowledge," don Juan Matus, whose descendants in this lineage, he said, went back ten thousand years. Aldous Huxley (author of *Brave New World*) made mescaline (the main psychoactive ingredient in peyote) familiar to the mainstream, with *The Doors of Perception* (1953), the title taken from the line by Blake: "If the doors of perception were cleansed, everything would appear to man as it is, Infinite." He took the drug under the supervision of British psychiatrist Humphrey Osmond. He wrote that "by 12:30 p.m., a vase of flowers becomes the 'miracle, moment by moment, of naked existence.'" Wikipedia summarizes his conclusions:

> Firstly, the urge to transcend one's self is universal through times and cultures (and was characterized by H. G. Wells as The Door in the Wall). [Huxley] reasons that better, healthier "doors" are needed than alcohol and tobacco. Mescaline has the advantage of not provoking violence in takers, but its effects last an inconveniently long time and some users can have negative reactions. Ideally, self-transcendence would be found in religion, but Huxley feels that it is

unlikely that this will ever happen. Christianity and mescaline seem well-suited for each other; the Native American Church for instance uses the drug as a sacrament, where its use combines religious feeling with decorum.

Huxley concludes that mescaline is not enlightenment or the Beatific vision, but a "gratuitous grace" (a term taken from Thomas Aquinas' *Summa Theologica*). It is not necessary but helpful, especially so for the intellectual, who can become the victim of words and symbols. Although systematic reasoning is important, direct perception has intrinsic value too. Finally, Huxley maintains that the person who has this experience will be transformed for the better.

MDMA

MDMA (Molly, Ecstasy) is not a plant, but this man-made molecule has therapeutic properties, particularly to the treatment of PTSD, and in its ability to help individuals clear their heart of negative past experiences. MDMA, a psychoactive drug, can give heightened sensations and euphoria. Typically, these effects last from three to six hours.[267] It is often classified as an "empathogen," as it helps individuals drop into a state of compassion, empathy and forgiveness, which gives it both therapeutic and social benefits. First synthesized in 1912, it was used by psychotherapists in the '70s but became illegal in 1985, as reckless use became prevalent.

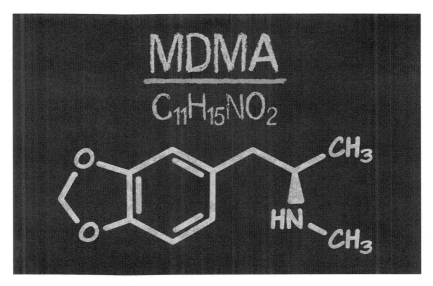

MDMA structure (Shutterstock)

Despite the setback in the '80s, MDMA is re-emerging in a new series of studies involving recovery from PTSD, autism, social anxiety, and more. In fact, in 2017 it was assigned a "breakthrough therapy designation" after the FDA reevaluated its potentially robust effect on PTSD. Over twenty veterans take their life daily, according to a VA study of data from 1979 to 2014. The suicide rate among veterans was 21 percent higher than among civilians.[268] These alarming numbers have been a wake-up call to the mental health community and the CDC to recognize that traditional pharmacotherapy and counseling are not cutting it, and that MDMA may offer a much greater therapeutic efficacy in halting this trend. A trial of MDMA-assisted psychotherapy for those with severe post-traumatic stress disorder is now in Phase 3.[269]

MDMA has been used extensively by the rave culture to enhance the heart connection to one another and induce a higher ecstatic state while dancing to electronic music. (See my interview with

Linda in the dance chapter.) Physical and psychiatric complications may occur in raves, especially with those who—to amplify the effects—create a cocktail of medications, psychedelics, and alcohol. This has led to hospitalizations and law-enforcement crackdowns. Increasing the risk of adverse effects and infrequently death, the purity of the compound is quite variable and in rare cases has been laced with fentanyl. While I have never participated in a rave, I have heard stories of amazing healing in these settings and understand the passion behind these gatherings. We can only hope that they can find a safe and legal way to do this in the future. As with all compounds discussed in this chapter, if you decide to work with one of these compounds, please proceed in a legal, safe setting and under the guidance of a therapist or skilled provider and with approval from your physician. Participating in a research trial using pharmaceutical-grade MDMA may be an option if you are currently suffering from PTSD.

Legalizing this drug for medicinal use and reintroducing this compound into the therapeutic setting, under the guidance of certified practitioners, with manufacturing by an FDA-approved facility, is the most rational, safe, and beneficial move forward legislatively. This would open the door for the deeper healing so needed amongst veterans and many other victims of violence. Using this compound therapeutically can help them release those retained traumas, open up their hearts and minds, and allow them to love others again. Numbing them with SSRIs, benzodiazepines, and narcotics may lead to more tragedies announced on the evening news.

LSD

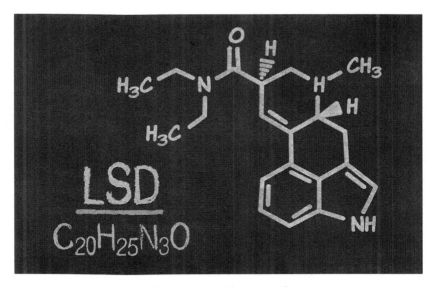

LSD structure (Shutterstock)

Although the LSD molecule is also not naturally occurring, it has a similar base structure to many plant medicines, and a prominent legal history in psychiatry in the 1950s, making it relevant for discussion. It helped scientists to better understand brain chemistry, thus pinning down the role of serotonin, which eventually led to the modern-day antidepressants, such as Prozac and Paxil. From a psychiatric research perspective, Czech psychiatrist Stanislav Grof in the 1970s said: *"Psychedelics, used responsibly and with proper caution, would be for psychiatry what the microscope is for biology and medicine or the telescope is for astronomy."*

In the 1950s while hallucinogenic drugs were legally available, pioneering psychiatrists like Humphrey Osmond and John Smythies tested their use in therapy—to treat alcoholism and several mental disorders—and were making headway until a backlash brought on the Controlled Substances Act, as mentioned earlier. Below, the *Guardian* reports on "A Brief History of Psychedelic Psychiatry":

> Between the years of 1950 and 1965, some 40,000 patients had been prescribed one form of LSD therapy or another as treatment for neurosis, schizophrenia, and psychopathy. It was even prescribed to children with autism. Research into the potential therapeutic effects of LSD and other hallucinogens had produced over 1,000 scientific papers and six international conferences
>
> Preliminary findings seemed to warrant further research into the therapeutic benefits of hallucinogenic drugs. The research soon came to an abrupt halt, however, mostly for political reasons. In 1962, the U.S. Congress passed new drug safety regulations, and the Food and Drug Administration designated LSD as an experimental drug and began to clamp down on research into its effects. The following year, LSD hit the streets in the form of liquid soaked onto sugar cubes; its popularity grew quickly and the hippy counterculture was in full swing by the summer of 1967.[270]

How was LSD discovered? LSD was first synthesized, by accident, in a laboratory by Swiss medicinal chemist Albert Hoffmann in 1938, while working for Sandoz Labs. It had been shelved for a number of years, but in April 1943, acting on a premonition, he decided to pull the dusty bottle off the shelf. After coming into contact with a small amount, and enjoying that serendipitous, mild experience, he was drawn to trying what he thought was still a small amount (but it wasn't)—just 250 micrograms, orally. Afterwards he had the wildest bike ride home imaginable. He said, "I perceived an uninterrupted stream of fantastic picture, extraordinary shapes with intense, kaleidoscopic play of colors.[271] About this famous incident much has been written:

> Hofmann had synthesized LSD in his lab as a medical stimulant for the respiratory and circulatory system in 1938, but at the time he didn't know what powers it held. Revisiting his discovery five years later, he caught a glimpse of its effects when some of the drug was absorbed through his fingertips, describing the experience as "dream-like" and a *"not unpleasant intoxicated-like condition."*
>
> Intrigued, three days later—on a day that would go down in history as "Bicycle Day"—he did what any responsible scientist would do: Experiment on himself.
>
> Taking a dose of 250 micrograms in his laboratory, thinking it was an appropriate threshold dose (we know now that he overdid it; 200 micrograms is the standard), Hofmann turned on, tuned in, and dropped out for the first time. Within an hour, his perception began to ebb and flow rapidly, and he began to freak out, convinced that his neighbor was a witch and that he was going insane. Hofmann wanted to go home.[272]

In the Amazon publicity for his memoir, *LSD: My Problem Child—Reflections on Sacred Drugs, Mysticism and Science,* he praises the role mystical experiences play in the planet's survival. "Whether induced by LSD, meditation, or arising spontaneously, such experiences help us to comprehend 'the wonder, the mystery of the divine, in the microcosm of the atom, in the macrocosm of the spiral nebula, in the seeds of plants, in the body and soul of people.'"

I feel John Lennon's lyrics and peaceful, compassionate demeanor were manifested partly by his psychedelic journeys with LSD, and other compounds that stimulated DMT.

This is best noted in his song "Imagine":

> You may say I'm a dreamer
> But I'm not the only one
> I hope someday you'll join us
> And the world will be as one

Whether his lyrics or the words of dreamers and leaders such as Martin Luther King and Mahatma Gandhi ring true to you, our survival is in part due to our human capacity to dream through our hearts, radiating this compassionate healing needed for modern society.

Bringing back these ancient healing plants, along with their synthetic counterparts, *in a legal, safe, controlled setting*, could have profound psychological effects both in individuals and society as a whole—rather than blunting unresolved traumas with mood stabilizers and antidepressants. Additionally, if these healing plants become normalized within Western society, the hatred and polarization found in modern society may ultimately trend towards greater compassion. As Gandhi said, "The day the power of love overrules the love of power, the world will know peace." Psychoactive plants may play a key role in realigning us with Gandhi's strength and connection to inner self and nature; to respect and love for others; and to oneness—these fundamental properties rippling out into the universe. Imagine the transformations that could arise from a facilitated Camp David retreat with the president and cabinet members using empathogenic plants to stimulate thought on world peace!!!

As we move towards this state of enlightenment with or without the use of these plant allies, we will activate DNA to help us make these quantum spiritual leaps for mankind.

Whether you decide to use psychoactive plants or compounds as part of your spiritual journey is fundamentally a personal decision and up to you. I am not encouraging you to do so but am providing this chapter to you for a broad-spectrum contemplation within the context of shifting your genome. Different options and paths work for different people, just as the same genetic pathway in two people can be turned on in one, off in the other, or be turned on and positive in one, turned on and negative in the other. The same even holds true for many medications I prescribe, such as high blood pressure medicines, asthma meds, and more. What works for one individual may have no effect or even an adverse effect on another.

In summary, the use of psychoactive plants and their synthetic relatives should follow these basic guidelines:

1. Consume it only in a country or state where it is legal, in an appropriate religious, research, and/or medical setting.

2. Seek the supervision of an experienced therapist, healthcare professional, or shaman who can monitor you during the journey and help you integrate and process it afterwards. Be aware, it can be difficult to assess the competency of shamans, since there are no certifications or overseeing boards; one has to research this through trusted local sources or agencies. In indigenous villages shamans are identified by consensus, not by self-proclaiming themselves as shaman.

3. Participate in a setting that is safe, reputable, sacred, and respectful to the plant medicine, recognizing that this is not a party, but a deep personal journey.

4. Always disclose your medications to the healer prior to ceremony, and if drug/plant interactions are noted, the medication should be discontinued prior to ceremony under the approval and guidance of your physician if possible, or one should avoid the ceremony.

5. Discussing plans with an integrative or functional-medicine physician or provider who is knowledgeable is also advised for further oversight/second opinion of possible drug interactions, medical, and psychiatric contraindications (e.g., bipolar, schizophrenia), or risks to your health based on a medical condition (i.e., heart/kidney/liver disease, etc.).

To summarize, the shamans of the ancient past and present are deep healers who play an ongoing role in their local community and facilitate the healing of others from around the world. Shamans, in fact—not the physicians of today—are the first functional-medicine healers. Modern functional medicine is the practice of treating the underlying root problem. Those functional-medicine providers who embrace shamanic healing apply not only modern-day tests and treatments, but also deploy a deep knowledge of natural healing with plants, herbs, nutrition, sound, and energy work.

I'm hopeful to see more modern-day healers experience, understand, and eventually integrate these options or refer interested patients who need this deeper work to safe and reputable therapists, shamanic practitioners, or retreat centers. Being open to collaborating beyond the evidence-based ivory halls of academia—to branch out like a balanced tree to the misty rays and healers in the emerald forests—will enable humankind to reconnect and heal emotionally, spiritually, mentally, and physically. Only then can we comprehensively and effectively promote the depth and breadth of epigenetic enhancement we once possessed.

Conclusion

Putting It All Together, Finding and Embracing "Oneness" in Your Life

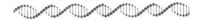

*The first peace, which is the most important,
is that which comes within the Souls of people
when they realize their relationship, their oneness
with the universe and all its powers, and when
they realize at the center of the universe dwells
the Great Spirit, and that its center is really
everywhere, it is within each of us.*

—Black Elk, Lakota medicine man.

As I was contemplating how to synthesize the concepts in the book, an event from five years ago came to mind, and the word "oneness" kept appearing in my field.

I remembered myself drumming in sacred circle with don Oscar Miro-Quesada near the base of Mount Shasta in northern California in 2013. As a reminder, Oscar is the originator of Peruvian Pachakuti Mesa Tradition cross-cultural shamanism and is an internationally acclaimed teacher and healer, an Earth-honoring ceremonialist. The circle was co-facilitated by Robert Vetter, a Native American anthropologist.

Following the opening of the circle, the approximately twenty of us began drumming together. The tempo of our primal beats started slow, then shifted, accelerating in an undulating manner. I could feel myself entering an altered state. Holding my elk hide shamanic hand drum, beating it with a padded stick, I noticed how my hand—outside my conscious control—began to synchronize and flow with the group, as if the universe was autopiloting it. Inside my trance state, I felt myself flowing and merging into this group.

As my mind quieted, I sensed a vortex of energy spiraling from our circle of drum beats, resonating into the cosmos. I felt Mother Earth underfoot and Father Sky coming through my crown to create an ecstatic state of timeless oneness. I had experienced this before, but the setting—in the beautiful circular ceremonial room—and group energy took me to a new level. Wow, I was blown away at how something as simple as drumming could do this!

The greatest goal of this book is to enlighten readers in ways to experience and embody oneness, which at the same time will impact DNA. Combining one or a few of the modalities discussed in this book should help you get there. While it would not be feasible to be in a state of continuous oneness in our modern-day lives, even experiencing it for a few seconds will help connect your heart to the infinite space, love, and compassion from the universe around you. Once you achieve this experience, you can share it and encourage others to find it as well. My guess is that many of you have already experienced it!

So what is "Oneness"? Is it just another esoteric New Age term or something legitimate and worthy of scientific exploration? Over thousands of years, much has been written on this concept, and theories around it are growing, particularly in astrophysics and cosmology.

Concepts contributing to the understanding of Oneness include the list below:

- Universal Consciousness or Universal Mind

- Unity Consciousness

- Cosmic Consciousness

- Quantum Consciousness

- Christ Consciousness

- Buddha nature, Nirvana

- The Law of One (source)

- Unified Field Theory (Einstein)

- Singularity Theory

- Nonduality Theory

- Quantum Field Theory

- Source Field

- Multidimensional connectivity

- Fractal and Sacred Geometry

- Holographic Universe

- Unus Mundus

Disciplines contributing to our expanded understanding of Oneness number among them:

- Theoretical physics

- Astrophysics

- Cosmology

- Particle physics

- Mathematics

- Fractal geometry, Sacred Geometry

- Biochemistry

- Study of light and sound

- Biology, neuroscience, genetics

- Religion and spirituality, particularly mysticism, Christ consciousness, Hinduism, Islam, and Buddhism.

- Sacred sexuality, Tantra

- Shamanism

- Psychedelic exploration of consciousness

- Exploration of the light body and luminous body

I consider this to be a short list of concepts and disciplines that make the deep dive into "Oneness." It's a topic worthy of volumes of books; I've seen hundreds listed on Amazon. My objective is to give you an overview to spark further investigations. For those that disagree with my views on Oneness, I embrace your opinion to agree, disagree, or further expand our understanding, working in this spirit of collective consciousness in a positive way! It may be beyond our human capacity to know the truth on Oneness, but as we continue this quest with the assistance of artificial intelligence, space exploration, and collaborative research amongst these disciplines, we may find the answers sooner than expected. Perhaps a unified theory between science and spirituality on this subject could help us find peace and greater ecological sustainability on this planet. Wolfgang Pauli addressed this unified theory, saying: "It would be most satisfactory of all if physis and psyche could be seen as complementary aspects of the same reality."

Regarding Jung, with whom Pauli discussed this theory, here is a little more of what he meant: "The unexpected parallelisms of ideas in psychology and physics suggest, as Jung pointed out, a possible ultimate oneness of both fields of reality that physics and psychology study. . . . The concept of a unitarian idea of reality (which has been followed up by Pauli and Erich Neumann) was called by Jung the *unus mundus* (the one world, within which matter and psyche and are not yet discriminated or separately actualized."[273]

Mentioned earlier in an interview with Kimba Arem, HeartMath's Global Coherence Initiative and the Global Consciousness Project (the latter originally directed by Roger Nelson, Coordinator of Research at the Princeton Engineering Anomalies Research, or PEAR, laboratory at Princeton University but with a logistics base currently at the Institute of Noetic Sciences) are attempting to put a finger on the pulse of our collective minds. HeartMath is utilizing sensors around the world to assess our "interconnectedness of human/animal health and behavior and the sun and earth's magnetic activity."[274] The Global Consciousness Project, utilizes a distributed network of random number generators to assess our emotional response to world events, from tragic tsunamis to the Academy awards.[275] Skeptics have created some controversy over their methodology and the technology of random number generators, but as long as they are true RNGs (TRNGs), generating random numbers from a physical process, not using algorithms, their results are impressive to many who have truly read the research.

What do others have to say on the perspectives of "Oneness"?

Finding Inner Alignment with Eckhart Tolle

Remembering that Eckhart Tolle, had written about it in *A New Earth: Awakening to Your Life's Purpose*, I searched my bookshelves and dusted off my copy, loaded with highlighted sentences from almost a decade ago. Tolle captured it well, saying:

> Inner alignment with the present moment opens your consciousness and brings it into alignment with the whole, of which the present moment is an integral part. The whole, the totality of life, then acts though you . . . But all things in existence, from microbes to human beings to galaxies, are not really separate things or entities, but form a web of interconnected multidimensional processes . . . Thinking cuts reality up into lifeless fragments . . . The whole is made up of existence and Being, the manifested and unmani-

fested, the world and God. So when you become aligned with the whole, you become a conscious part of the interconnectedness of the whole and its purpose: the emergence of consciousness into this world. Nature exists in a state of unconscious oneness with the whole.[276]

Later he asserts the importance of being ego free, quoting Jesus: "Blessed are the meek, for they shall inherit the Earth." Tolle feels, "The meek are the egoless. They live in the surrendered state and so feel their oneness with the whole and the Source."[277] I am hopeful that we can shift the mindset of our ego-inflated leaders to a more balanced or ego-free state, rather than run the risk of seeing them destroy our world, sending us back again to a primal survival state. Our leaders might have the capacity to let go of ego, but in this position of power and control, it is unlikely they will relinquish ego for the greater good.

Opening Your Heart and Connecting to Oneness

It all begins by making a habit of practicing leading with our hearts, raising our energy, and tuning in to greater information and frequencies of love and wholeness....The future of humanity does not rest on one person, leader, or messiah with a greater consciousness to show us the way. Rather it requires the evolution of a new collective consciousness, because it is through the acknowledgement and the application of interconnectedness of human consciousness that we can change the course of history.[278]

—Joe Dispenza

Researching the climaxes of highly advanced ancient civilizations—during my travels to places such as Caral, Peru; Luxor, Egypt; the Temples of Delos Island, Greece; the Uxmal Maya temples in Yucatan; Easter Island, and many more—has been enlightening. While visiting a site, one has to experience the artwork, geometry, and energy, rather than simply reading or listening to an archeological and historical interpretation. Meditating at these sites in a quiet area has brought in the deepest insights. My sense is that these civilizations peaked during a matriarchal period or time when the Divine Feminine prevailed over the masculine. They embraced a more ego-free state and a more compassionate and supportive society. Their downfall typically occurred when leaders dove too aggressively into masculine pursuits of conquest rather than balancing those pursuits with nurturing their homeland.

Perspectives on Freeing the Mind and Going Inward

If you want oneness in society, you have to teach people to go inside instead of going outside, because if they want peace, they need to find it within.

—Ram Dass

The universe is not outside of you. Look inside yourself; everything that you want, you already are.

—Rumi

I'm trying to free your mind, Neo. But I can only
show you the door. You're the one that has to walk
through it.

—Morpheus in the movie *The Matrix*

Ram Dass, Rumi, and Morpheus show us the door to going inward, thus finding a greater understanding of the mystery that surrounds us. It is up to us to limit or eliminate our addiction to TVs, computers, and smartphones to foster a more meaningful reconnection to our inner self. By doing this, we will be freer from materialism and politics, less distracted from this inner work. If we lack the will, our suffering will continue.

I read the above Ram Dass quote to my daughter today at the dinner table. She's currently pursuing a major in environmental science and replied saying, "To go inside, sometimes we have to go outside, Dad."

"Exactly," I replied. "Hiking or meditating in nature allows me to do more inward work, but it's not so easy to do in the chaos and fragmented energy of a city." We agreed that many of our contemporary nation's leaders, having minimal to no connection with nature, unfortunately see it as something to be exploited. Maybe a multiday hike in the woods, beyond the trails at a Camp David retreat, is what's really needed for many of them.

Connecting to the Holographic and Vibratory Universe

> We are beginning to see the entire universe as a holographically interlinked network of energy and information. We and all things in the universe are nonlocally connected with each other and with all other things in ways that are unfettered by the hitherto known limitations of space and time.
>
> —Ervin Laszlo, Hungarian philosopher and
> Integral theorist

Visionary artist Alex Grey expands further, saying, "The infinite vibratory levels, the dimensions of interconnectedness are without end. There is nothing independent. All being are residents in our oneness."[279] So, much of his art connects through oneness and love, offering a visual perspective that can be appreciated well in normal consciousness or an altered state.

In my conversation with author, channel, and spiritual adventurer Jonette Crowley, she describes her experience like this: "I most often connect to universal consciousness by meditating, though sometimes it happens spontaneously at any time. When it happens, it is the feeling of soft bliss. It is a space beyond words and surprisingly emotionless, except for a deep feeling of endless well-being. I want to stay there forever, but if I try too hard, I'll fall out of the state. It puts the rest of my life in perspective, because in this state, you know that bliss is the only reality."

Going to a Place of Love

If I go into the place in myself that is love and you go into the place in yourself that is love we are together in love. Then you and I are truly in love, the state of being love. That's the entrance to Oneness. That's the space I entered when I met my guru.

—Ram Dass

Unifying Science and Spirituality

The day science begins to study the non-physical phenomena, it will make more progress in one decade than in all previous centuries of existence.

—Nikola Tesla

Sacred Sexuality—Fostering Oneness

I touched on the topic of sacred sexuality earlier, but feel it deserves a final comment regarding its importance in experiencing oneness. Someday, I'll attempt to write a separate book on this subject!

Experiencing oneness with a partner during orgasm can be an out-of-body experience, creating a deep sacred-sexuality union. The loving spiraling of kundalini energies from root to crown, followed by the orgasmic expansion into the universe together or sequentially, is one of the most powerful things we can feel. The ecstasy and the flow of Shakti dissolves our ego as we let go, traveling into this interdimensional space of oneness. As Melissa Eisler, author and meditation instructor, explains: "Shakti, one of the most important goddesses in the Hindu pantheon, is really a divine cosmic energy that represents feminine energy and the dynamic forces that move through the universe."[280] We have to let go of our egos to achieve this state of ecstasy and connection—let go and surrender to what we are doing, naturally flowing and sensing the spiraling of sexual energies.

For those without partners, this can be experienced with self-pleasure as one similarly sets an intention to flow and let go into oneness. One can go there, however, by flowing into a heart-centered state with or without a partner, and without the need to involve sexuality. Surrendering openheartedly to a place of compassion, self-love, and love for others can take you there.

Ken Cohen, in *The Way of Qigong*, touches on this principle: "Qigong relaxation skills also increase sensitivity to sexual needs and our capacity to surrender to the sexual experience." He feels that Dan Tian (hara: centered in the belly) breathing is helpful in enhancing jing (bodily fluids) and sexual energy.[281] I feel the practice of tantra, qigong, and other ancient traditions can guide us further in our intimate relationships, as long as we don't get too distracted by the technique, which risks separating us from the flow.

In *Eros Ascending: The Life Transforming Power of Sacred Sexuality*, John Maxwell Taylor summarizes: "When we practice sacred sexuality, we are working with cosmologically rooted principles, balancing the heavenly yang (male energy) of the universe with the all-knowing, life-giving yin (feminine energy) of the earth within ourselves."[282]

I'm hopeful to see a shift from within the religious community that will embrace sacred sexuality in a way that facilitates reaching an individual's soul connection to oneness and the god within, rather than pushing outdated doctrines that ultimately repress sexuality, preventing deeper personal development and more intimate relationships.

Now that I have briefly overviewed the concepts of oneness, I hope this will help you discover some of the various strategies discussed in this book that you didn't know about to optimally shift your DNA and that of those around you. Experiencing even transient states of oneness can be life changing. Are there ways to combine meditation, sound healing, and other methods so as to make these quantum leaps? If so, how can we do this while at the same time staying grounded enough to maintain our daily routines?

Everyone will have a unique answer. For me, sometimes it's simply drumming or hiking alone in a mountain forest, sensing the energy and sacred geometry of the trees and ferns. Other times it may happen as I gaze at the dome of infinite stars with plant medicine and music.

Perhaps spinning like a dervish will get you there; or a trip to a Peruvian jungle, with the exotic sounds of the rain forest during an ayahuasca journey, is needed. Most of us will need to try various mindful-based modalities to find the key or keys to unlocking the oneness experience.

Most importantly, I encourage readers to venture boldly and diversely to find those unique keys. Always keep safety in mind, seeking out experts and a safe setting to guide you on the deeper work. Experiment by alchemizing elements such as sound therapy, breathwork, sacred geometry, and even dance to help unlock the deeper you! Over time, you'll discover and resonate with things I didn't mention, that will shift you even more profoundly opening more doors. As you find your personal formula, diving deeper and deeper, you will have more moments of spiritual awakening and insights. This may motivate you to make a sacred pilgrimage to Mount Kailash or simply to connect with a friend over coffee. Exotic or seemingly mundane, each step could lead to another quantum shift. Friends, places, and experiences will catalyze you. Temples and pyramids will shift you, as will meditating with a Buddhist monk. Giving you this unique guide to opportunities will hopefully increase your thirst for spiritual adventure beyond a yoga class or an all-inclusive beach vacation in Mexico.

Synchronicities will increase as you travel, and more opportunities will become available as you expand your web of connections to like-minded individuals. The synchronicities in my life have grown so exponentially that it's become difficult to keep track of them! I want them to explode for you too.

I'm not a guru, and simply see myself as another human being seeking enlightenment. I see myself as a modern healer integrating the wisdom of ancient medicine and spirituality to help others on their path. Where I am at on the path depends in part on where we as a whole are on this path. By helping others, we create an interlaced unified field of spiritual growth. So as I send light and ideas into the fabric of universal consciousness, I hope you will weave your own beautiful pattern to blend in as well. Connect to the woven interdimensional pattern meditatively and resonate with the colors that amplify your prana or qi. As you breathe this in, amplify it and share it out to heal others. Clear any dark energies or negativity by flowing white light or rainbow light energy through your body. Again, what resonates with you may be something entirely different than what I've presented, and that's fine. I'm just hopeful that whatever path you choose, you seek light, not darkness, and envision a growing web of higher-resonate beings, interlinked to preserve our existence on this fragile planet.

I wish you success in your quest to find oneness, ecstasy, and ultimately greater love and compassion for one another. As others become awakened through this work, their DNA will epigenetically shift as a result of increased happiness and reductions in stress. This will bring ultimately greater health and longevity, and an ability to contribute more to a healthier planet and society. Most of what has manifested in this book came in beyond my 3-D world, from the multidimensional, 4-D and higher. I have added scientific evidence in regard to epigenetics (changing your DNA) to support many concepts, but a lot of what I've discussed will require much more sophisticated technology to discover the secrets of our highly complex multidimensional universe.

Society will objectively classify me in one box or another, but my goal is to free myself and my ideas beyond our primitive, egoic human and artificial-intelligence filing cabinets. We are way more than a racial description, professional title, political affiliation, Wikipedia listing, Google search, or social-media post. We are a drop in the ocean of universal consciousness that is timeless and expansive—our drop in this life, past and future, that will continue to expand and permeate the field of the entire universe. We have a choice of sending light and sacred geometry or darkness and chaos into our drops. I'm hopeful you will choose the first, regardless of your religion or spiritual pursuits.

If we simply choose love, compassion, and forgiveness, our course is set in the right direction. When we do so, our DNA responds, resonating with this woven pattern of rainbow light, bringing health and ongoing awakening into the higher dimensions of space, time, oneness, and beyond . . . Wishing all of you an amazing life that connects you to love and healing of the multiverse surrounding you!

Acknowledgments

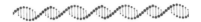

I am thankful for all the support and help I received while writing this book. Especially to my wife Theresa, daughter Brooke, and son Keaton. Also, to my parents, who encouraged me along the way and have been lifetime role models, emphasizing service to others above self. So much gratitude goes out to my editor, Margaret A. Harrell, who helped me maintain momentum and provided amazing editorial assistance throughout this long journey. Thanks to KA'ryna SH'ha for finding such a beautiful way to capture the essence of this book in the cover art and Darlene Swanson for her book formatting and design.

Gratitude for spiritual insights brought by my circle of friends in meditation and shamanic groups, including Jonette Crowley, Terry Smith, Miguel Angel, Kelly Roberts, James Loan, Jyoti Stewart, Cydney Fodeman, Daniel Frank, Kim Miller, Melissa Kade, Gurpreet Kaur, Darlene Joy, and many others. Thank you to don Oscar Miro-Quesada, Garry Caudill, and Paula Givan, who taught me the Pachakuti Mesa tradition, and to the all mesa holders around the world, including Tiffany Binder and Shelly Genovese. Gratitude to sacred geometers Greg Hoag and Francene Hart and the insights of Drunvalo Melchizedek. Frequency and vibrational gratitude to sound healers Jonathan

351

Goldman, Kimba Arem, and Ron Minson, and to John Stuart Reid's depth of knowledge on the geometry of sound known as cymantics. Thank you to Jef Crab, Elizabeth Wilcock, Sharon Wehner, and Linda Driscoll-Powers, who have provided us with the keys to flowing vital energy through our bodies through qigong, ballet, and dance. Thanks to Austyn Lewis, my amazing office manager, for keeping my medical office running efficiently and for volunteering to be featured in the sound-healing photos. My apologies if I missed anyone!

Thank you to Gaia (Mother Earth), who has nurtured and sustained us all but must also be nurtured back. Last but not least, thank you to my patients, who for over twenty-six years have been foundational in teaching me how to listen and heal in an opened-minded, heart-centered way to the infinite possibilities within and beyond the halls of modern medicine.

Notes

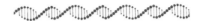

Chapter 1:

1   Robert Bartz, "Remembering the Hippocratics," in Bioethics: *Ancient Themes in Contemporary Issues*, 4.

2   "Asclepius and the Temples of Healing," http://www.historywiz.com/didyouknow/asclepius.html.

3   "Temple of Asclepius, Rome," Wikipedia, https://en.wikipedia.org/wiki/Temple_of_Asclepius,_Rome.

4   David K. Osborn, "Greek Medicine," http://www.greekmedicine.net/whos_who/Hippocrates.html.

5   Jacques Jouanna, *Hippocrates*, 16.

6   Emma J. and Ludwig Edelstein, *Asclepius: Interpretation of the Testimonies*, reprint 1998, Johns Hopkins, https://jhupbooks.press.jhu.edu/content/asclepius.

7   Jouanna, *Hippocrates*, 4, 27.

8   "History," International Hippocratic Foundation of Kos, http://hippocraticfoundation.org/the-institution/history.

9   Jouanna, *Hippocrates*, 12.

10   Mark Cartwright, "Asclepius," *Ancient History Encyclopedia*, https://www.ancient.eu/Asclepius.

11   Cartwright, "Kos," *Ancient History Encyclopedia*, https://www.ancient.eu/Kos/; also Wikipedia, "Cyparissus," https://en.wikipedia.org/wiki/Cyparissus," and "Asclepeion of Kos," Kos Island, Greece (website), https://www.kos4all.com/4899/asclepeion-of-kos/.

12   Vivian Nutton, *Ancient Medicine*, 2nd ed., 53–54.

13 Nutton, *Ancient Medicine*, 70.

14 Jouanna, *Hippocrates*, 17.

15 Jouanna, *Hippocrates*, 10.

16 Jouanna, *Hippocrates*, 27.

17 "The Asklepieion, Reconstruction Drawing and Plan" (after Stuart Rossiter, *Blue Guide Greece*, London 1977, 660–662), https://www.ostia-antica. org/kos/asklep-p/asklep-p.htm.

18 Spyros G. Marketos, "History of Medicine," http://asclepieion.mpl.uoa. gr/Parko/marketos2.htm.

19 Nutton, *Ancient Medicine*, 114.

20 "Asclepieia—The Health Centers of Antiquity," http://www.grethexis. com/asclepeia-health-centers-antiquity/.

21 Nutton, *Ancient Medicine*, 110.

22 "The Kos Castle of the Knights," Greek Islands Post Cards (website), http://www.greekisland.co.uk/kos/sights/knights-castle.html.

23 "Decline of the Colosseum," Roman Empire & Colosseum (website), http://www.tribunesandtriumphs.org/colosseum/decline-of-the-colos-seum.htm. Also see James Lees-Milne, *Saint Peter's—The Story of Saint Peter's Basilica in Rome*. London: Hamish Hamilton, 1967. Referenced in Wikipedia, "St. Peter's Basilica": Pope Nicholas V (1447–'55) "had, however, ordered the demolition of the Colosseum and by the time of his death, 2,522 cartloads of stone had been transported for use in the new building," https://en.wikipedia.org/wiki/St._Peter%27s_Basilica.

24 Nutton, *Ancient Medicine*, 87.

25 "World Population," Wikipedia.

26 Thomas P. Duffy, "The Flexner Report—100 Years Later," *Yale Journal of Biology and Medicine* 84, no. 3 (Sept. 2011), 269–76, https://www.ncbi. nlm.nih.gov/pmc/articles/PMC3178858/.

27 Carl Jung, *Symbols and the Interpretation of Dreams*, Collected Works 18, par. 585.

28 Jerry W. Swanson, "Vitamin D and MS: Is There Any Connection?" http:// www.mayoclinic.org/diseases-conditions/multiple-sclerosis/expert-an-swers/vitamin-d-and-ms/faq-20058258.

29 Mark Jeschke, "Weed Management in the Era of Glyphosate Resistance," https://www.pioneer.com/home/site/us/agronomy/weed-mgmt-and-glyphosate-resis/.

30 Organic Consumers Association, "Monsanto Is Putting Normal Seeds Out of Reach," https://www.organicconsumers.org/news/monsanto-putting-normal-seeds-out-reach.

31 Carey Gillam, "Roundup Herbicide Research Shows Plant, Soil Problems," https://www.reuters.com/article/us-glyphosate/roundup-herbicide-research-shows-plant-soil-problems-idUSTRE77B58A20110812.

32 Ruth Bender, "Bayer Hit by More Lawsuits over Safety of Roundup Weed Killer," https://www.wsj.com/articles/bayer-hit-by-more-lawsuits-over-safety-of-roundup-weedkiller-1542098262.

33 Marshall Allen, "How Many Die from Medical Mistakes in U.S. Hospitals?" https://www.scientificamerican.com/article/how-many-die-from-medical-mistakes-in-us-hospitals/.

34 "Monsanto Merger . . . or Bust?" http://www.panna.org/blog/monsanto-merger-or-bust.

35 Jay C. Fournier et al., "Antidepressant Drug Effects and Depression Severity: A Patient-Level Meta-analysis." *JAMA* 303, no. 1 (2010): 47–53.

36 "*Guns, Germs, and Steel,*" Wikipedia.

37 Melissa Denchak, "Paris Climate Agreement: Everything You Need to Know," Dec. 18, 2018, https://www.nrdc.org/stories/paris-climate-agreement-everything-you-need-know.

Chapter 2:

38 Marshall Allen, "How Many Die from Medical Mistakes in U.S. Hospitals?" https://www.scientificamerican.com/article/how-many-die-from-medical-mistakes-in-us-hospitals/.

39 Bruce Lipton, *The Biology of Belief: Unleashing the Power of Consciousness, Matter and Miracles,* 137–38.

40 Elissa Epel et al., "Can Meditation Slow Rate of Cellular Aging? Cognitive Stress, Mindfulness, and Telomeres?" *Annals of the New York Academy of Sciences* 1172 (Aug. 2009): 34–53, https://doi.org/10.1111/j.1749-6632.2009.04414.x.

41 T. L. Jacobs et al, "Intensive Meditation Training, Immune Cell Telomerase Activity, and Psychological Mediators. *Psychoneuroendocrinology* 36, no. 5 (June 2011): 664–81.

42 Shiv Basant Kumar et al., "Telomerase Activity and Cellular Aging Might Be Positively Modified by a Yoga-Based Lifestyle Intervention," *The Journal of Alternative and Complementary Medicine* 21, no. 6 (June 2015): 370–72.

43 Quinn Conklin et al., "Telomere Lengthening after Three Weeks of an Intensive Insight Meditation Retreat," *Psychoneuroendocrinology* 61 (Nov. 2015): 26–27.

44 E. S. Epel et al., "Accelerated Telomere Shortening in Response to Life Stress," *Proceedings of the National Academy of Sciences of the United States of America* 101, no. 49 (2004), 17312–315, https://www.ncbi.nlm.nih.gov/pmc/articles/PMC534658/.

45 Carmen Martin-Ruiz et al., "Telomere Length Predicts Poststroke Mortality, Dementia, and Cognitive Decline," http://onlinelibrary.wiley.com/doi/10.1002/ana.20869/abstract.

46 Masood A. Shammas, "Telomeres, Lifestyle, Cancer, and Aging," https://www.ncbi.nlm.nih.gov/pmc/articles/PMC3370421/.

47 Adam G. Marsh, Matthew T. Cottrell, and Morton F. Goldman, "Epigenetic DNA Methylation Profiling with MSRE: A Quantitative NGS Approach Using a Parkinson's Disease Test Case," *Frontiers in Genetics* (Nov. 2, 2016), https://doi.org/10.3389/fgene.2016.00191.

48 Flora Carr, "Scott Kelly Spent a Year in Space and Now His DNA Is Different from His Identical Twin's," *Time* magazine, http://time.com/5201064/scott-kelly-mark-nasa-dna-study/.

49 Michelle Corey, "Methylation: Why It Matters for Your Immunity, Inflammation & More," https://www.mindbodygreen.com/0-18245/methylation-why-it-matters-for-your-immunity-inflammation-more.html,

50 David S. Black and George M. Slavich, "Mindfulness Meditation and the Immune System: A Systematic Review of Randomized Controlled Trials," *Annals of the New York Academy of Sciences* 1373, no. 1 (June 2016): 13–24, doi: 10.1111/nyas.12998.

51 Michelle Ye Hee Lee, "The Missing Context behind the Widely Cited Statistic That There Are 22 Veteran Suicides a Day," Fact Checker *Washington Post*, https://www.washingtonpost.com/news/fact-checker/wp/2015/02/04/the-missing-context-behind-a-widely-cited-statis-

tic-that-there-are-22-veteran-suicides-a-day/?noredirect=on&utm_
term=.9ba6e5209fc2.

52 Grof Transpersonal Training (website), "About Holotropic Breathwork,"
http://www.holotropic.com/holotropic-breathwork/about-holotropic-
breathwork/.

Chapter 3:

53 Robert Lawlor, *Sacred Geometry: Philosophy & Practice*, 16.

54 "Pythagorean Theorem," Wikipedia.

55 *Convivialium disputationum*, liber 8, 2; quoted in "Sacred Geometry,"
Wikipedia.

56 Lawlor, *Sacred Geometry*, 6.

57 Vitruvius, *De Architectura*, Book V, Ch. 4.8. Translation. 8. "These have
taken their names from numbers. For when the voice has rested in one
fixed sound, and then modulates and changes from itself, and comes
to the fourth sound it is called diatessaron; when it comes to the fifth,
it is called diapente; to the eighth, diapason; to the eleventh, diapason
with diatessaron; to the twelfth, diapason with diapente to the fifteenth
disdiapason," http://www.vitruvius.be/boek5h4.htm.

58 Gordon Plummer, *The Mathematics of the Cosmic Mind*. Quoted by Robert
Lawlor. *Sacred Geometry* (1982), 96. Sourced in the article "309ct
3-D20-Icosahedron-Real Amethyst Quartz Gemstone #213." https://
rjrockshop.com/products/309ct-3-d20-icosahedron-real-amethyst-
quartz-gemstone-hand-carved-213?variant=581238685709.

59 Jean-Pierre Luminet et al., "Dodecahedral Space Topology as an
Explanation for Weak Wide-Angle Temperature Correlations in the
Cosmic Microwave Background," *Nature* 425 (Oct. 2003): 593.

60 Amanda Gefter, "Is the Universe a Fractal?' https://www.newscientist.
com/article/mg19325941-600-is-the-universe-a-fractal/.

61 Bruce Lipton, *The Biology of Belief*, 216.

62 Token Rock founders/contributors, "Flower of Life," http://www.token-
rock.com/explain-flower-of-life-46.html.

63 BBC UK, "Where I Live Wiltshire," Sept. 24, 2014 (archived), http://
www.bbc.co.uk/wiltshire/moonraking/spooky_leylines.shtml.

64 "What Is a 'Henge' Monument?" http://www.orkneyjar.com/history/
henge.htm.

65 English Heritage website, "History of Stonehenge," https://www.english-heritage.org.uk/visit/places/stonehenge/history-and-stories/history/.

66 Hillary Leung, "Stonehenge's Rocks Have Been Traced to Two Quarries 180 Miles Away," updated Feb. 21, 2019, http://time.com/5534188/stonehenge-bluestone-quarries-180-miles-away/.

67 Mike Parker Pearson et al, "Megalith Quarries for Stonehenge's Bluestones," *Antiquity* 93, no. 367 (Feb. 2019): 45–62, https://doi.org/10.15184/aqy.2018.111.

68 Freddy Silva, The Prophets Conference, http://www.greatmystery.org/nl/salisbury09geometry.html.

69 Austin Kinsley, "Restorations at Stonehenge," Oct. 1, 2017, https://www.silentearth.org/restorations-at-stonehenge-2/.

70 Maria Dasi Espuig, "Stonehenge Secrets Revealed by Underground Map," BBC News (Sept. 10, 2014), https://www.bbc.com/news/science-environ-ment-29126854.

71 Ed Caesar, "What Lies beneath Stonehenge?" https://www.smithsonian-mag.com/history/what-lies-beneath-Stonehenge-180952437/#Qu2Al1mAuLtSxim6.99.

72 "Research on Stonehenge," English Heritage website, http://www.english-heritage.org.uk/visit/places/stonehenge/history/research/.

73 Deborah Byrd, "Summer Solstice at Stonehenge," http://earthsky.org/earth/gallery-the-summer-solstice-as-seen-from-stonehenge.

74 Laura Geggel, "'German Stonehenge' Yields Grisly Evidence of Sacrificed Women and Children," June 28, 2018, https://www.livescience.com/62939-german-stonehenge-human-sacrifices.html.

75 UNESCO World Heritage site, "Dacian Fortresses of the Orastie Mountains," https://whc.unesco.org/en/list/906/.

76 What-When-How: In Depth Tutorials and Information (website), "Sarmizegetusa Regis," http://what-when-how.com/ancient-astronomy/sarmizegetusa-regia/.

77 Chiriac C. Nicolae and Alina Dragomir, "Dacians and the Great Sanctuary at Sarmizegetusa/the Dacian Calendar," March 5, 2018, https://www.matrixdisclosure.com/dacians-sanctuary-sarmizegetusa-calendar/.

78 Painton Cowen and Jill Purce, *Rose Windows*.

79 "A Flickering Light," Wezit Research Group, http://www.clinic.visnsoft.com/video1.htm.

80   "The Experience," PandoraStar (website), https://pandorastar.co.uk/intro-duction.

81   Anne Trafton, "Unique Visual Stimulation May Be New Treatment for Alzheimer's," http://news.mit.edu/2016/visual-stimulation-treatment-alzheimer-1207.

82   "Historical Introduction," Alhambra de Granada (website), https://www.alhambradegranada.org/en/info/historicalintroduction.asp.

83   Barbara O'Brien, "Mount Meru in Buddhist Mythology," updated July 24, 2017, https://www.thoughtco.com/mount-meru-449900.

84   Graham Hancock, *Heaven's Mirror: Quest for the Lost Civilization*, 126–127.

85   Natalie Wolchover, "A Jewel at the Heart of Quantum Physics," https://www.quantamagazine.org/20130917-a-jewel-at-the-heart-of-quantum-physics/.

86   Morihei Ueshiba, *The Art of Peace,* Shambhala Pocket Library Series, 5.

Chapter 4:

87   Leslie Taylor, "Rainforest Facts: The Disappearing Rainforests," http://www.rain-tree.com/facts.htm#.WmONzWcY7BU.

88   "Monteverde, Costa Rica," Monteverde Travel Guide (website), http://www.monteverdeinfo.com/.

89   Sidney B. Smith, "Fibonacci Sequence," *Platonic Realms Interactive Mathematics Encyclopedia,* http://platonicrealms.com/encyclopedia/Fibonacci-sequence.

90   Gary B. Meisner, "Phi/ What is the Fibonacci Sequence (aka Fibonacci Series)?" https://www.goldennumber.net/fibonacci-series/.

      Stephanie Pappas, "Human Body Part That Stumped Leonardo da Vinci Revealed," https://www.livescience.com/20157-anatomy-drawings-leonardo-da-vinci.html.

91   Euclid, "Euclid's *Elements*," Book VI, Definition 3, https://mathcs.clarku.edu/~djoyce/elements/bookVI/defVI3.html.

92   Pappas, "Human Body Part That Stumped Leonardo da Vinci Revealed," https://www.livescience.com/20157-anatomy-drawings-leonardo-da-vinci.html.

93   "*New World Encyclopedia* contributors, "Luca Pacioli," http://

www.newworldencyclopedia.org/p/index.php?title=Luca_Pacioli
&oldid=1013453 (revisions as of Aug. 2, 2018); they drew as well from
"Luca Pacioli," Wikipedia.

94 "Luca Pacioli," Wikipedia.

95 Meisner, "Life/Human Hand and Foot," http://www.goldennumber.
net/human-hand-foot/.

96 Matthew Cross and Robert Friedman, Introduction, *The Golden Ratio &
Fibonacci Sequence*, 10.

97 Meisner, "Life/DNA Spiral as a Golden Section," http://www.golden-
number.net/dna/.

98 Caroline Myss, "The Seven Chakras," https://www.myss.com/free-re-
sources/world-religions/hinduism/the-seven-chakras/.

99 Cross and Friedman, Introduction, *The Golden Ratio & Fibonacci
Sequence*.

100 Richard Cassaro, "Occult Secrets behind Pine Cone Art & Architecture,"
https://www.richardcassaro.com/occult-symbolism-behind-pine-cone-
art-architecture/.

101 NASA online, "The Milky Way Galaxy, https://imagine.gsfc.nasa.gov/
science/objects/milkyway1.html.

102 Francene Hart, *Sacred Geometry of Nature*, 51.

103 "Sacred Geometry," Seed of Life Institute, http://www.solischool.org/
sacred-geometry.html.

104 Stephen S. Hall, "Hidden Treasures in Junk DNA," https://www.scien-
tificamerican.com/article/hidden-treasures-in-junk-dna/.

105 Princeton University, "Imaging in Living Cells Reveals How 'Junk
DNA' Switches on a Gene," *ScienceDaily*, July 23, 2018, http://www.
sciencedaily.com/releases/2018/07/180723142817.htm.

106 Aaron Rowe, "Diamonds 'Entangled' in Physics Feat," http://lightyears.
blogs.cnn.com/2011/12/07/diamonds-entangled-in-physics-feat/.

107 Pete Wilton, "Vibration Rocks for Entangled Diamonds," Dec. 16,
2011, https://phys.org/news/2011-12-vibration-entangled-diamonds.
html#jC.p.

108 Nassim Haramein, "The I-Ching Encodes the Geometry of the Fabric
of Space-Time," https://www.facebook.com/Nassim.Haramein.official/
videos/286050751586190/.

109 Haramein Facebook page, https://www.facebook.com/Nassim. Haramein.official/. February 12, 2018, at 3:22 p.m

Chapter 5:

110 Paramahansa Yogananda (website), "Excerpts from *God Talks with Arjuna: The Bhagavad Gita by Paramahansa Yogananda*," http://yoga-nanda.com.au/gita/gita0614om.html.

111 Annaliese and John Stuart Reid, "Sound Healing—Ancient Sounds," https://www.tokenrock.com/sound_healing/sounds_of_the_ancients/, content courtesy of the Reids, copyright © 2011, http://www.cymas-cope.com/. Also see A. J. Block, "What Is a Didgeridoo (the Droning Aboriginal Australian Wind Instrument)?" Oct. 28, 2015, https://didgeproject.com/free-didgeridoo-lessons/what-is-a-didgeridoo/.

112 Annaliese and J. S. Reid, ''Sound Healing—Ancient Sounds."

113 As quoted on "Sound Healing—Ancient Sounds," http://www.token-rock.com/sound_healing/sounds_of_the_ancients/, content courtesy of John Stuart and Analiese Shandra Reid, © 2011, http://www.cymas-cope.com.

114 Vandana Mohata, "Mantras: An Interview with Jonathan Goldman," https://www.healingsounds.com/mantras-an-interview-with-jonathan-goldman/.

115 Email from John Stuart Reid to the author March 14, 2019. My great thanks to Reid, who was instrumental in reviewing and submitting content for the following paragraphs on his work.

116 John Stuart Reid et al., "What is Cymatics?" https://www.cymascope.com/cyma_research/index.html.

117 Reid et al., "The Science of the CymaScope," http://www.cymascope.com/cymascope.html.

118 Mandara Cromwell and John Stuart Reid, "What's That? (Part One) with ISTA's Mandara Cromwell," http://www.cymaticsconference.com/wordpress/wp-content/uploads/2017/10/DIY-Cymatics-with-JSR.pdf.

119 John Stuart Reid et al., "Cymatics Research—Biology: The Shape of Life, We Believe, Is Sound," https://www.cymascope.com/cyma_re-search/biology.html.

120 Email from John Stuart Reid to the author March 14, 2019.

121 Reid et al., "Cymatics Research—Biology."

122 Amy Novotney, "Music as Medicine," sourced at American Psychological Association website, http://www.apa.org/monitor/2013/11/music.aspx.

123 Andrea Rossi et al., "Music Reduces Pain Perception in Healthy Newborns: A Comparison between Different Music Tracks and Recorded Heartbeat." *Early Human Development* 124 (2018): 7–10.

124 Jonathan Goldman, "The Humming Effect: The Simplest Sound Is the Most Profound," Aug. 17, 2017, https://www.soundhealersassociation. org/blog/139-the-humming-effect-the-simplest-sound-is-the-most-profound-2017-by-jonathan-goldman.html.

125 T. M. Gilmor, "The Tomatis Method and the Genesis of Listening," *Journal of Prenatal & Perinatal Psychology & Health* 4, no. 1 (1989): 9–26.

126 See "Alfred Tomatis" under "Discover" on the Tomatis website, https:// www.tomatis.com/en.

127 The Monroe Institute website, https://www.monroeinstitute.org/.

128 So Sound quotation, http://www.sosoundsolutions.com/products/so-sound-mattress/.

129 F. H. Rauscher, G. L. Shaw, and Katherine N. Ky, "Music and Spatial Task Performance," Nature 365 (Oct. 14, 1993): 611 (research article that spawned the Mozart-effect book). Also see J. S. Jenkins, "The Mozart Effect," *Journal of the Royal Society of Music* 94, no. 4 (April 2001): 170–72), https://www.ncbi.nlm.nih.gov/pmc/articles/PMC1281386/.

130 Rauscher et. al., "Music and Spatial Task Performance: A Causal Relationship," presented at the American Psychological Association 102nd Annual Convention, Los Angeles, Aug. 12–16, 1994, sourced at http://www.burchschool.com/music-and-spatial-task-performance-a-causal-relationship/.

131 Esperanza M. Anaya, David B Pisoni, and William G Kronenberger, "Visual Spatial-Sequence Learning and Memory in Trained Musicians," *Psychology of Music* 45, no. 1 (2017): 19.

132 "Research Update on the Sound Techniques of Cymatechnologies: The Cyma 1000 Cymatechnologies Device Successfully Trialed on Thoroughbred Racehorses," https://cymatechnologies.com/sound-from-ancient-roots/sound-therapy-articles/research-update-on-the-sound-techniques-of-cymatechnologies/. Also see E. B. Bauer et al., "The Effects of Acoustic Frequencies on Core Tendon Lesions of the Thoroughbred Racehorse," https://cymatechnologies.com/wordpress/wp-content/uploads/2014/08/Tendon-Lesion-Repair.pdf.

133 See "So Sound Solutions," http://www.sosoundsolutions.com/products/so-sound-treatment-tables/. Also see PandoraStar UK (website), https://pandorastar.co.uk. Also, "Researching the Human Heart and Brain," the HeartMath Institute, https://www.heartmath.org/research/.

134 Innovative Medicine, "About Pulsed Electromagnetic Field Therapy," https://innovativemedicine.com/solutions/pulsed-electromagnetic-field-therapy/.

135 Kimba Arem, "Music as Medicine," http://gaearth.com/.

136 "Secret of Water—The Movie," www.secretofwaterthemovie.com.

137 Lund University, "Dolphins Use Double Sonar: Researchers Discover That Dolphins Can Generate Two Sound Beam Projections Simultaneously," *ScienceDaily*, 8 June 2011, https://www.sciencedaily.com/releases/2011/06/110607112338.htm; Edwina Shaw, "Science Shows Dolphins Communicate Holographically," Dec. 1, 2016, https://upliftconnect.com/dolphins-communicate-holographically/.

138 Reid et al., "First 'What-the-dolphin-saw' Image of a Submerged Man: Cymatic-Holographic Imaging Technique," http://www.cymascope.com/cyma_research/oceanography.html; Jack Kassewitz et al., "A Phenomenon Discovered While Imaging Dolphin Echolocation Sounds," Journal of Marine Science: Research & Development, July 15, 2016, https://www.omicsonline.org/open-access/a-phenomenon-discovered-while-imaging-dolphin-echolocation-sounds-2155-9910-1000202.php?aid=76570.

139 Annette Deyhle, "Earth's Atmosphere, Schumann Resonance, and the Ionosphere."

140 Gregg Braden, "Magnetic Field, Schumann Resonance, Pole Shift, and 2012," https://www.bing.com/videos/search?q=Greg+Braden%2c+schumann+frequencies&qpvt=Greg+Braden%2c+schumann+frequencies&view=detail&mid=808900F567FC31C8C137808900F567FC31C8C137&&FORM=VRDGAR.

141 Justin Deschamp, "HeartMath Institute: The Schumann Resonances Are Not Rising," May 13, 2017, on *Stillness in the Storm*, http://www.stillnessinthestorm.com/2017/05/heartmath-institute-the-schumann-resonances-are-not-increasing.html.

142 The National Institute of Mental Health and Neuroscience in India supports the benefits of chanting and humming. See Bangalore G. Kalyani et al., "Neurohemodynamic Correlates of 'Om' Chanting," *International Journal of Yoga* 4, no. 1 (2011): 3–6, http://yogafordepression.com/wp-content/uploads/Neurohemodynamic-correlates-of-'OM'-chanting.pdf.

143 Don Campbell, *The Mozart Effect: Tapping the Power of Music to Heal the Body, Strengthen the Mind, and Unlock the Creative Spirit*, New York: William Morrow, 2001.

Chapter 6:

144 Masaru Emoto, *The Secret Life of Water*, Atria paperback, 178.

145 Wallace J. Nichols, *Blue Mind: The Surprising Science That Shows How Being Near, In, On, or Underwater Can Make You Happier, Healthier, More Connected, and Better at What You Do*, 203.

146 "The Adventure of Discovery," http://www.fabiencousteauolc.org/.

147 Wikiquotes, from *Time* (March 28, 1960).

148 BC Whales (website), "Humpback Whale Song," https://www.bcwhales.org/humpback-whale-song/.

149 N. J. Saunders, *Animal Spirits*, 25.

150 Environmental News Network Staff, "Dolphins Studied for Pollution's Impact," Feb. 4, 1999, http://www.cnn.com/TECH/science/9902/04/dolphins.enn/.

151 Bruce E. Becker, "Healing Waters," *Aquatics International* (June 1, 2007), 27–32.

152 Richard G. Hunter, "Epigenetic Effects of Stress and Corticosteroids in the Brain," *Frontiers in Cellular Neuroscience* 6 (2012): 18.

153 Hassan Khasbek et al., "The Role of Water H-Bond Imbalances in B-DNA Substrate Transitions and Peptide Recognition Revealed by Time-Resolved FTIR Spectroscopy," *Journal of the American Chemical Society* 133, no. 15 (March 2011): 5834–42.

154 Emoto, *The Secret Life of Water*, 183.

155 Goldman, *The 7 Secrets of Sound Healing*, 40.

156 Emoto, *The Secret Life of Water*, 71–102.

157 Dieter Kunz et al., "A New Concept for Melatonin Deficit: on Pineal Calcification and Melatonin Excretion," *Neuropsychopharmacology* 21, no. 6 (Jan. 2000): 765–72; Jennifer Luke, "Fluoride Deposition in the Aged Human Pineal Gland," *Caries Research* 35, no. 2 (2001): 125–28. Research has also shown a link between pineal gland calcification and Alzheimer's.

158 "Mount Shasta," in *Picturesque California* (1888–1890), 165; reprinted in *Steep Trails* (1918), Chapter 5; sourced in "John Muir," Wikiquotes.

159 Emoto, in an excerpt from *The Secret Life of Water*, https://www.dailyom.com/cgi-bin/display/librarydisplay.cgi?lid=2530.

Chapter 7:

160 Gloria A. Young, "Sun Dance," Encyclopedia of Oklahoma History and Culture. The Oklahoma Historical Society, http://www.okhistory.org/publications/enc/entry.php?entry=SU008.

161 Young, "Sun Dance."

162 "The American Indian Religious Freedom Act 1978," University of Idaho website, http://www.webpages.uidaho.edu/~rfrey/329AIRFA.htm.

163 Paul U. Unschuld, *Medicine in China: A History of Ideas*, Berkeley: University of California Press, 1985.

164 Jef Crab's website: www.jefcrab.com.

165 Elizabeth Wilcock, in conversation.

166 Sol Luckman, "All Healing Is Really Self-Healing," https://www.tokenrock.com/articles/all-healing-is-really-self-healing/. Article adapted from the author's *Potentiate Your DNA: A Practical Guide to Healing & Transformation with the Regenetics Method*.

167 Emoto, *The Secret Life of Water*.

168 "Original Research Discoveries" (of Glen Rein), Innovative Biophysical Technologies, http://www.innobioteck.com/discoveries.html.

169 "Rein, "Effect of Conscious Intention on Human DNA."

170 Tori Rodriguez, "Descendants of Holocaust Survivors Have Altered Stress Hormones," March 1, 2015, https://www.scientificamerican.com/article/descendants-of-holocaust-survivors-have-altered-stress-hormones/.

171 Adam Klosin et al., "Transgenerational Transmission of Environmental Information in C. Elegans," *Science* 356, no. 6335 (April 2017): 320–23, https://doi.org/10.1126/science.aah6412.

172 Michael Winn, "Curing Cancer Naturally with Chi Kung," http://www.healingcancernaturally.com/medical-qigong-cancer-therapy.html.

173 Winn, "Curing Cancer Naturally with Chi Kung [Qigong] Self-Healing Therapy."

174 Marlowe and Company.

175 Paul Dong and Aristide H. Esser, *Chi Gong: The Ancient Chinese Way to Health*, 1990. See also Dr. Mark Sircus, "Carpet Bombing Cancer with Invincible Oxygen" (Feb. 11, 2014), http://drsircus.com/general/carpet-bombing-cancer-with-invincible-oxygen/.

176 Sankara Subramanian, "Adumu: The traditional Maasai Dance," Oct. 5, 2012, https://www.beontheroad.com/2012/10/adumu-traditional-maasai-dance.html#.

177 "Rumi and the Whirling Dervishes," Facts and Details, http://factsanddetails.com/world/cat55/sub394/item1436.html.

178 "Sama (Sufism)," Wikipedia.

179 Bruce Finley, "It's Not Your Imagination: More Trees Than Ever Are Standing Dead in Colorado Forests," Feb. 15, 2017, https://www.denverpost.com/2017/02/15/dead-trees-colorado-forests/.

180 BBC News, "Ancient 'Massacre' Unearthed Near Lake Turkana, Kenya," Jan. 21, 2016, https://www.bbc.com/news/world-africa-35370374.

181 Khaliya, "The Promise of Ecstasy for PTSD," https://www.nytimes.com/2017/11/03/opinion/ecstasy-ptsd.html.

182 S. S. Jiao et al., "Brain-derived Neurotrophic Factor Protects against Tau-related Neurodegeneration of Alzheimer's Disease," *Translational Psychiatry* 6, no. 10 (Oct. 4, 2016): e907, https://doi.org/10.1038/tp.2016.186.

183 "About Us," Dance for PD, https://danceforparkinsons.org/about-the-program.

184 Kathrin Rehfeld et al., "Dancing or Fitness Sport? The Effects of Two Training Programs on Hippocampal Plasticity and Balance Abilities in Healthy Seniors." *Frontiers in Human Neuroscience* 11 (June 15, 2017): 305. Accessed online at "Dancing Can Reverse the Signs of Aging in the Brain," *ScienceDaily* 25 (Aug. 2017). www.sciencedaily.com/releases/2017/08/170825124902.htm. https://www.frontiersin.org/articles/10.3389/fnhum.2017.00305/full.

185 Rehfeld et al., "Dancing or Fitness Sport?"

186 Rehfeld et al., "Dancing or Fitness Sport?"

187 Joe Verghese et al., "Leisure Activities and the Risk of Dementia in the Elderly," *New England Journal of Medicine* 348 (Jan. 19, 2003): 2508–16, https://doi.org/10.1056/NEJMoa022252.

188 Richard Powers, "Dancing Makes You Smarter," https://socialdance. stanford.edu/syllabi/smarter.htm.

189 Janissa Delzo, "Improve Brain Function by Playing Super Mario and Other Video Games, Science Says," *Newsweek* online (Dec. 7, 2017), http://www.newsweek.com/improve-brain-function-playing-super-ma-rio-and-other-video-games-science-says-741592.

190 Holly Hammond, "The Timeline and History of Yoga in America" (Aug. 29, 2007), http://yogajournal.com/yoga-101/yogas-trip-america.

Chapter 8:

191 Stephen Kotler and Jamie Wheal, *Stealing Fire*, 2–3

192 Kotler, "Exploring the Intersection between Radical Innovation, Peak Performance, & Disruptive Technology," http://www.stevenkotler.com/.

193 Orrin Devinsky et al., "Trial of Cannabidiol for Drug-Resistant Seizures in the Dravet Syndrome," *New England Journal of Medicine*, 376 (May 25, 2017): 2011–20, https://doi.org/10.1056/NEJMoa1611618.

194 Sean Markey, "CBD Bioavailability: What's the Best Way to Absorb CBD?" July 31, 2018, updated Oct. 19, https://www.cannahealth.org/cbd-bioavailability-whats-the-best-way-to-absorb-cbd/.

195 "Cannabinoids Remove Plaque-forming Alzheimer's Proteins from Brain Cells: Preliminary Lab Studies at the Salk Institute Find THC Reduces Beta Amyloid Proteins in Human Neurons" (June 27, 2016), https://www.salk.edu/news-release/cannabinoids-remove-plaque-form-ing-alzheimers-proteins-from-brain-cells/.

196 Sanjay Gupta, "Weed 4: Pot vs. Pills," CNN transcript of April 29, 2018.

197 Thomas Brown, "Observational Study of the Long-Term Efficacy of Ibogaine-Assisted Therapy (Mexico)," https://maps.org/ibogaine-ther-apy-for-drug-addiction/170-observational-study-of-the-long-term-effi-cacy-of-ibogaine-assisted-therapy-mexico.

198 National Institute on Drug Abuse, "Overdose Death Rates" (rev. Jan. 2019), https://www.drugabuse.gov/related-topics/trends-statistics/over-dose-death-rates.

199 Centers for Disease Control and Prevention (CDC), "Fact Sheets—Alcohol Use and Your Health," https://www.cdc.gov/alcohol/fact-sheets/alcohol-use.htm.

200 Karen Cullen et al., "Use of Electronic Cigarettes and Any Tobacco Product among Middle and High School Students—United States, 2011–2018," CDC *Morbidity and Mortality Weekly Report* (*MMWR*), 67, no. 45: 1276–77, https://www.cdc.gov/mmwr/volumes/67/wr/mm6745a5.htm?s_cid=mm6745a5_w.

201 Master Teacher, "Drug Harm Charts and Psychedelics," *Cognitive Liberty—UK*, https://cognitivelibertyuk.wordpress.com/2011/08/09/drug-harm-charts-psychedelics/.

202 NIH, "Prescription Opioid Use Is a Risk Factor for Heroin Use," https://www.drugabuse.gov/publications/research-reports/relationship-between-prescription-drug-heroin-abuse/prescription-opioid-use-risk-factor-heroin-use.

203 Biljana Bauer Petrovska, "Historical Review of Medicinal Plants' Usage," *Pharmacognosy Reviews* 6, no. 11 (Jan.–June 2012): 1–5, https://doi.org/10.4103/0973-7847.95849.

204 David Hill, "Peru's Ayahuasca Industry Booms as Westerners Search for Alternative Healing" (Jan. 7, 2016), https://www.theguardian.com/travel/2016/jun/07/peru-ayahuasca-drink-boom-amazon-spirituality-healing.

205 NIH, "Alcohol Facts and Statistics," https://www.niaaa.nih.gov/alcohol-health/overview-alcohol-consumption/alcohol-facts-and-statistics.

206 Martin Boroson, Martin Duffy, and Barbara Egan, "Healing and Transformation: The Use of Non-Ordinary States of Consciousness," https://iahip.org/inside-out/issue-13-summer-1993/healing-and-transformation-the-use-of-non-ordinary-states-of-consciousness.

207 Javier Regueiro, *San Pedro Huachuma*, 2017, 15.

208 Regueiro, *San Pedro Huachuma*, 11.

209 Regueiro, *San Pedro Huachuma*, 204.

210 Vaults of Erowid, "Walter Pahnke. Jan. 18, 1931–July 10, 1971," https://erowid.org/culture/characters/pahnke_walter/pahnke_walter.shtml.

211 Kotler and Wheal, *Stealing Fire*, 50.

212 "A Brief History of Psychedelic Psychiatry," *The Guardian*, U.S. edition, Sept. 2, 2014, https://www.theguardian.com/science/neurophilosophy/2014/sep/02/psychedelic-psychiatry.

213 Lance Dodds and Zachary Dodds, "The Sober Truth: Debunking the Bad Science behind the 12-Step Program and the Rehab Industry," http://sobertruthbook.com/.

214 Patrick Smith, "What Is the Legality of Ayahuasca in Your Home?" (Jan. 18, 2017), https://thethirdwave.co/legality-ayahuasca/.

215 CDC, "Fatal Injury Reports: National, Regional and State, 1981–2016," https://webappa.cdc.gov/sasweb/ncipc/mortrate.html.

216 "Data Brief 241: Increase in Suicide in the United States, 1999–2014 and Data Table for Figure 1. Age-Adjusted Suicide Rates, by Sex: United States, 1999–2014," https://www.cdc.gov/nchs/data/databriefs/db241_table.pdf. Retrieved Nov. 2017.

217 "Suicide." National Institute of Mental Health. Retrieved Sept. 8. 2017.

218 J. C. Fournier et al., "Antidepressant Drug Effects and Depression Severity: A Patient-Level Meta-Analysis," *Journal of the American Medical Association* 303, no. 1 (2010): 47–53, https://doi.org/10.1001/jama.2009.1943.

219 J. M. Ferguson, "SSRI Antidepressant Medications: Adverse Effects and Tolerability," *Primary Care Companion to The Journal of Clinical Psychiatry* 3, no. 1 (2001): 22–27.

220 AØ Bielefeldt, P. B. Danborg, and P. C. Gøtzsche. "Precursors to Suicidality and Violence on Antidepressants: Systematic Review of Trials in Adult Healthy Volunteers," *Journal of the Royal Society of Medicine* 109 (2016): 381–92, https://doi.org/10.1177/0141076816666805.

221 National Institute on Drug Abuse, "Overdose Death Rates" (rev. Jan. 2019), https://www.drugabuse.gov/related-topics/trends-statistics/over-dose-death-rates.

222 "Gun Violence Archives: Past Summary Ledgers—Archives 2014–2018, http://www.gunviolencearchive.org/past-tolls.

223 Aaron Karp, "Estimating Global Civilian-Held Firearms Numbers," Briefing Paper 2018, http://www.smallarmssurvey.org/fileadmin/docs/T-Briefing-Papers/SAS-BP-Civilian-Firearms-Numbers.pdf.

224 Elizabeth Chuck, "Is Social Media Contributing to Rising Teen Suicide Rate?" Oct. 22, 2017, https://www.nbcnews.com/news/us-news/social-media-contributing-rising-teen-suicide-rate-n812426.

225 Mayo Clinic Staff, "Selective Serotonin Reuptake Inhibitors (SSRIs)," May 17, 2018, https://www.mayoclinic.org/diseases-conditions/depression/in-depth/ssris/art-20044825.

226 David Plans, "We've lost Touch with Our Bodies," Feb. 5, 2019, https://blogs.scientificamerican.com/observations/weve-lost-touch-with-our-bodies.

227 Kate Wheeling, "Bio Tech Company Marks Up Drug Cost by 5,000 Percent Because It Can," Sept. 22, 2015, https://psmag.com/economics/biotech-company-marks-up-drug-cost-by-5000-percent-because-it-can.

228 Reuters (NBC News), "Bernie Sanders Asks Why Drug, Once Free, Now Costs $375,000," Feb. 4, 2019, https://www.nbcnews.com/politics/2020-election/bernie-sanders-asks-why-drug-once-free-now-costs-375-n966746.

229 Matthew Herper (Forbes staff), "David Graham on the Vioxx Verdict," Aug. 19, 2005, https://www.forbes.com/2005/08/19/merck-vioxx-graham_cx_mh_0819graham.html#7251a0835698.

230 Subash, C. Gupta, Sridevi Patchva, and Bharat B. Aggarwal, "Therapeutic Roles of Curcumin: Lessons Learned from Clinical Trials," *Journal of the American Association of Pharmaceutical Scientists* 15, no. 1 (Jan. 2013): 195–218, https://doi.org/10.1208/s12248-012-9432-8.

231 American Heart Association, "Fish and Omega-3 Fatty Acids," Last reviewed March 23, 2017, http://www.heart.org/HEARTORG/HealthyLiving/HealthyEating/HealthyDietGoals/Fish-and-Omega-3-Fatty-Acids_UCM_303248_Article.jsp#.WmzQdJM-dR0.

232 Michael Aviram and Mira Rosenblat, "Pomegranate for Your Cardiovascular Health," *Rambam Maimonides Medical Journal* 4, no. 2 (April 2013): e0013, https://doi.org/10.5041/RMMJ.10113.

233 Andrew Jacobs, "Opposition to Breast-Feeding Resolution by U.S. Stuns World Health Officials" (July 8, 2018), https://www.nytimes.com/2018/07/08/health/world-health-breastfeeding-ecuador-trump.html.

234 "Dr. Albert Einstein Dies in Sleep at 76: World Mourns Loss of Great Scientist," *New York Times* obituary (April 19, 1955), 35.

235 Source for number of Amazon plant species. K. Morales, and T. Vinicius, "Amazon Rainforest: Biodiversity and Biopiracy," *Student BMJ*, no. 13 (2003): 386–87.

236 Jeremy Narby, *The Cosmic Serpent: DNA and the Origins of Knowledge*, 92–93.

237 Fred Grover, "Lumerian Crystal Map," https://www.google.com/maps/d/u/0/edit?mid=1VoTUIhMr9oICvtjSI6WbkC1GgK0&ll=7.391949464929354%2C0&z=2.

238 Joshua Eagle, "3 Powerful Tools for Pineal Gland Activation," https://wakeup-world.com/2015/04/04/the-3-most-powerful-tools-for-pineal-gland-activation/

239 Bianca Garilli, "MTHFR Mutation: A Missing Piece in the Chronic Disease Puzzle," *Holistic Primary Care* 13, no. 2 (June 18, 2012), https://holisticprimarycare.net/topics/topics-a-g/functional-medicine/1353-mthfr-mutation-a-missing-piece-in-the-chronic-disease-puzzle.html.

240 Rick Strassman, *DMT: The Spirit Molecule*, 42.

241 Alexander Shulgin and Ann Shulgin, *Tihkal* (1997), 247–84.

242 Strassman, *The Spirit Molecule*, 55.

243 Strassman, *The Spirit Molecule*, 52.

244 Strassman, *The Spirit Molecule*, 52.

245 Puakai: Healing through the Energy of Mother Nature (website), https://puakaihealing.com/model/.

246 K. Mandrake, *The Psilocybin Mushroom Bible: The Definitive Guide to Growing and Using Magic Mushrooms.*

247 Christian Orlic, "The Origins of Directed Panspermia" (Jan. 9, 2013), https://blogs.scientificamerican.com/guest-blog/the-origins-of-directed-panspermia/.

248 Terence McKenna, "The Stoned Ape Theory," https://www.youtube.com/watch?v=ZnEKoFrx1rI.

249 Paul Seaburn, "The Return of the Stoned Ape Theory of Evolution" (July 27, 2017), http://mysteriousuniverse.org/2017/07/the-return-of-the-stoned-ape-theory-of-evolution/.

250 Robin McKie, "Interview—Colin Blakemore: How the Human Brain Got Bigger by Accident and Not Through Evolution," https://www.theguardian.com/technology/2010/mar/28/colin-blakemore-how-human-brains-got-bigger.

251 "Marsh Chapel Experiment," based on Wikipedia: version of Oct. 13, 2016. https://ipfs.io/ipfs/QmXoypizjW3WknFiJnKLwHCnL72vedxjQkDDP1mXWo6uco/wiki/Marsh_Chapel_Experiment.html.

252 Roland Griffiths et al., "Mystical-Type Experiences Occasioned by Psilocybin Mediate the Attribution of Personal Meaning and Spiritual Significance 14 Months Later," *Journal of Psychopharmacology* 22, no. 6 (Aug. 2008): 621–32, https://doi.org/10.1177/0269881108094300.

And Roland Griffiths et al., "Psilocybin Can Occasion Mystical Type Experiences Having Substantial and Sustained Personal Meaning and Spiritual Significance," *Psychopharmacology* 187, no. 3 (Aug. 2006): 268–83, https://doi.org/doi: 10.1007/s00213-006-0457-5.

253   Griffiths et al., "Mystical-Type Experiences Occasioned by Psilocybin."

254   Griffiths et al., "Psilocybin Produces Substantial and Sustained Decreases in Depression and Anxiety in Patients with Life-Threatening Cancer," *Journal of Psychopharmacology* 30, no. 12 (2016), 1181–97, http://journals.sagepub.com/doi/pdf/10.1177/0269881116675513.

255   Michael Pollan, *How to Change Your Mind*, 77.

256   G. Petri et al., "Homological Scaffolds of Brain Functional Networks," Dec. 6, 2014, https://doi.org/10.1098/rsif.2014.0873.

257   Kevin Loria, "How Psychedelics like Psilocybin and LSD Actually Change the Way People See the World," *Business Insider*, Feb. 26, 2017, https://www.businessinsider.com/a-new-understanding-film-shows-how-psilocybin-changes-perception-2017-2.

258   Pollan, *How to Change Your Mind*, 125.

259   H. R. El-Seedi et al., "Prehistoric Peyote Use: Alkaloid Analysis and Radiocarbon Dating of Archaeological Specimens of Lophophroa from Texas," https://doi.org/10.1016/j.jep.2005.04.022.

260   J. Richard Andrews, *Workbook for the Introduction to Classical Nahuatl*, 246.

261   Richard Evans Schultes, "The Appeal of Peyote (Lophophora Williamsii) as a Medicine," *American Anthropologist* 40, no. 4 (1938): 698–715, http://www.samorini.it/doc1/alt_aut/sz/schultes_pey.htm.

262   Schultes and Albert Hofmann, "The Tracks of the Little Deer," from *Plants of the Gods: Their Sacred, Healing and Hallucinogenic Powers* (1992), https://www.peyote.org/.

263   Schultes, "The Appeal of Peyote (Lophophora Williamsii) as a Medicine," http://www.samorini.it/doc1/alt_aut/sz/schultes_pey.htm.

264   "Francisco Hernández de Toledo," Wikipedia.

265   Schultes, "The Appeal of Peyote (Lophophora Williamsii) as a Medicine."

266   Cultural Survival Inc., "Huichol," *Cultural Survival Quarterly Magazine* (June 1992), https://www.culturalsurvival.org/publications/cultural-survival-quarterly/huichol.

267 J. S. Meyer, "3,4—Methylenedioxymethamphetamine (MDMA): Current Perspectives," *Substance Abuse and Rehabilitation* 4 (Nov. 21, 2013): 83–99.

268 Leo Shane III and Patricia Kime, "New VA Study Finds 20 Veterans Commit Suicide Each Day," *Military Times*, https://www.militarytimes. com/veterans/2016/07/07/new-va-study-finds-20-veterans-commit-suicide-each-day/.

269 MAPS, "A Phase 3 Program of MDMA-Assisted Psychotherapy for the Treatment of Severe Posttraumatic Stress Disorder (PTSD)," https:// maps.org/research/mdma/ptsd/phase3.

270 "A Brief History of Psychedelic Psychiatry," *The Guardian*, U.S. ed. (Sept. 2, 2014), https://www.theguardian.com/science/neurophiloso-phy/2014/sep/02/psychedelic-psychiatry.

271 Albert Hoffmann, *LSD: My Problem Child*, 1980:15.

272 Yasmin Tayag, "On 'Bicycle Day,' Albert Hofmann Took the First LSD Trip," April 19, 2017, https://www.inverse.com/article/14503-bicycle-day-albert-hofmann-lsd-acid-trip.

Conclusion:

273 Thomas J. McFarlane, "Quantum Physics, Depth Psychology, and Beyond" (rev. June 21, 2000), http://www.integralscience.org/psyche-physis.html.

274 HeartMath Institute website, "Global Coherence Initiative," March 23, 2009, https://www.heartmath.org/articles-of-the-heart/global-intercon-nectedness/global-coherence-initiative/.

275 The Global Consciousness Project, "Introduction to GCP," http://noo-sphere.princeton.edu/gcpintro.html.

276 Eckhart Tolle, *A New Earth: Awakening to Your Life's Purpose*, 275–77.

277 Tolle, *A New Earth*, 309.

278 Joe Dispenza, *Becoming Supernatural: How Common People Are Doing the Uncommon*, 320–21.

279 Alex Gray, "Alex Gray Quotations," https://www.quotetab.com/quotes/by-alex-grey#gLOGDqbMByMbx0WS.97.

280 Editors at Chopra.com, "Shakti: A Universal Force," https://chopra.com/article/shakti-universal-force.

281 Kenneth S. Cohen, *The Way of Qigong: The Art and Science of Chinese Energy Healing*, 320.

282 J. M. Taylor, *Eros Ascending: The Life Transforming Power of Sacred Sexuality*, 48.

Works Cited

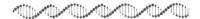

Alhambra de Granada (website). "Historical Introduction." https://www.al-hambradegranada.org/en/info/historicalintroduction.asp.

Allen, Marshall. "How Many Die from Medical Mistakes in U.S. Hospitals?" September 20, 2013. https://www.scientificamerican.com/article/how-many-die-from-medical-mistakes-in-us-hospitals/.

American Heart Association. "Fish and Omega-3 Fatty Acids." Last reviewed March 23, 2017. http://www.heart.org/HEARTORG/HealthyLiving/HealthyEating/HealthyDietGoals/Fish-and-Omega-3-Fatty-Acids_UCM_303248_Article.jsp#.WmzQdJM-dR0.

Anaya, Esperanza M., David B Pisoni, and William G Kronenberger. "Visual-Spatial Sequence Learning and Memory in Trained Musicians." *Psychology of Music* 45, no. 1 (2017): 5–21.

Andrews, J. Richard. *Workbook for the Introduction to Classical Nahuatl.* rev. ed. Norman, OK: University of Oklahoma Press, 2003.

Arem, Kimba. "Music as Medicine." http://gaearth.com/.

"Asklepieion, Reconstruction Drawing and Plan, The." After S. Rossiter, *Blue Guide Greece*, London, 1977. http://www.ostia-antica.org/kos/asklep-p/asklep-p.htmhttps://www.ostia-antica.org/kos/asklep-p/asklep-p.htm.

Aviram, Michael, and Mira Rosenblat. "Pomegranate for Your Cardiovascular Health." *Rambam Maimonides Medical Journal* 4, no. 2 (April 2013): e0013. Published online April 30, 2013. https://www.ncbi.nlm.nih.gov/pmc/articles/PMC3678830/.

Bartz, Robert. "Remembering the Hippocratics: Knowledge, Practice, and Ethos of Ancient Greek Physician-healers." In *Bioethics: Ancient Themes in Contemporary Issues,* edited by Mark G. Kuczewski and Ronald Polansky. Cambridge, MA: MIT Press, 2000.

BBC News. "Ancient 'Massacre' Unearthed Near Lake Turkana, Kenya." January 21, 2016. https://www.bbc.com/news/world-africa-35370374.

BBC UK. "Where I Live Wiltshire." September 24, 2014 (archived). http://www.bbc.co.uk/wiltshire/moonraking/spooky_leylines.shtml.

BC Whales (website)."Humpback Whale Song." https://www.bcwhales.org/humpback-whale-song/.

Becker, Bruce E. "Healing Waters." *Aquatics International* magazine (June 1, 2007): 27–32. Online at https://www.aquaticsintl.com/facilities/healing-waters-1_o.

Bender, Ruth. "Bayer Hit by More Lawsuits over Safety of Roundup Weed Killer." https://www.wsj.com/articles/bayer-hit-by-more-lawsuits-over-safety-of-roundup-weedkiller-1542098262.

Bielefeldt, A.Ø., P. B. Danborg, and P. C. Gøtzsche. "Precursors to Suicidality and Violence on Antidepressants: Systematic Review of Trials in Adult Healthy Volunteers." *Journal of the Royal Society of Medicine* 109 (2016): 381–392.

Black, David S., and George M. Slavich. "Mindfulness Meditation and the Immune System: A Systematic Review of Randomized Controlled Trials." *Annals of the New York Academy of Sciences* 1373, no. 1 (June 2016): 13–24. doi: 10.1111/nyas.12998.

Block, A. J. "What Is a Didgeridoo (the Droning Aboriginal Australian Wind Instrument)?" October 28, 2015. https://didgeproject.com/free-didgeridoo-lessons/what-is-a-didgeridoo/.

Boroson, Martin, Martin Duffy, and Barbara Egan. "Healing and Transformation: The Use of Non-Ordinary States of Consciousness." https://iahip.org/inside-out/issue-13-summer-1993/healing-and-transformation-the-use-of-non-ordinary-states-of-consciousness.

Braden, Gregg. "Gregg Braden, Magnetic Field, Schumann Resonance, Pole Shift, and 2012." YouTube. https://www.bing.com/videos/search?q=Greg+Braden%2c+schumann+frequencies&qpvt=Greg+Braden%2c+schumann+frequencies&view=detail&mid=808900F567FC31C8C137808900F567FC31C8C137&&FORM=VRDGAR.

Brown, Thomas. "Observational Study of the Long-Term Efficacy of Ibogaine-Assisted Therapy (Mexico)." https://maps.org/ibogaine-therapy-for-drug-addiction/170-observational-study-of-the-long-term-efficacy-of-ibogaine-assisted-therapy-mexico.

Byrd, Deborah. "Summer Solstice at Stonehenge." In Earth | Human World | June 19, 2018. http://earthsky.org/earth/gallery-the-summer-solstice-as-seen-from-stonehenge.

Caesar, Ed. "What Lies beneath Stonehenge?" https://www.smithsonianmag.com/history/what-lies-beneath-Stonehenge-180952437/.

Campbell, Don. *The Mozart Effect: Tapping the Power of Music to Heal the Body, Strengthen the Mind, and Unlock the Creative Spirit.* New York: Harper Collins/William Morrow, 2001.

Carr, Flora. "Scott Kelly Spent a Year in Space and Now His DNA Is Different from His Identical Twin's." *Time* magazine. Updated March 15, 2018 5:50 PM ET. http://time.com/5201064/scott-kelly-mark-nasa-dna-study/.

Cartwright, Mark. "Asclepius." *Ancient History Encyclopedia.* June 20, 2013. https://www.ancient.eu/Asclepius.

___. "Kos." *Ancient History Encyclopedia.* April 18, 2016. https://www.ancient.eu/Kos/.

Cassaro, Richard. "Occult Secrets behind Pine Cone Art & Architecture." December 19, 2010. https://www.richardcassaro.com/occult-symbolism-behind-pine-cone-art-architecture/.

Centers for Disease Control and Prevention (CDC). "Data Brief 241: Increase in Suicide in the United States, 1999–2014 and Data Table for Figure 1. Age-adjusted suicide rates, by sex: United States, 1999–2014." https://www.cdc.gov/nchs/data/databriefs/db241_table.pdf. Retrieved November 2017.

——. "Fact Sheets—Alcohol Use and Your Health." https://www.cdc.gov/alcohol/fact-sheets/alcohol-use.htm.

——. "Fatal Injury Reports: National, Regional and State, 1981–2016." https://webappa.cdc.gov/sasweb/ncipc/mortrate.html.

Chuck, Elizabeth. "Is Social Media Contributing to Rising Teen Suicide Rate?" October 22, 2017. https://www.nbcnews.com/news/us-news/social-media-contributing-rising-teen-suicide-rate-n812426.

Cohen, Kenneth S. *The Way of Qigong: The Art and Science of Chinese Energy Healing.* New York: Ballantine, 1999.

Conklin, Quinn, Brandon King, Anthony Zanesco, and Jen Pokorny. "Telomere Lengthening after Three Weeks of an Intensive Insight Meditation Retreat." *Psychoneuroendocrinology* 61 (2015): 26–27.

Corey, Michelle. "Methylation: Why It Matters for Your Immunity, Inflammation & More." https://www.mindbodygreen.com/0-18245/methylation-why-it-matters-for-your-immunity-inflammation-more.html.

Cowen, Painton, and Jill Purce. *Rose Windows*. San Francisco: Chronicle Books, 1979.

Crab, Jef. www.jefcrab.com.

Cromwell, Mandara, and John Stuart Reid. "What's That? (Part One) with ISTA's Mandara Cromwell." http://www.cymaticsconference.com/wordpress/wp-content/uploads/2017/10/DIY-Cymatics-with-JSR.pdf.

Cross, Matthew, and Robert Friedman. *The Golden Ratio & Fibonacci Sequence: Golden Keys to Your Genius, Health, Wealth & Excellence*. New Canaan, CT: Hoshin Media, 2013. Kindle.

Cullen, Karen A., Bridget K. Ambrose, Andrea S. Gentzke, Benjamin J. Apelberg, Jamal Ahmed, and Brian A King. "Use of Electronic Cigarettes and Any Tobacco Product among Middle and High School Students—United States, 2011–2018." CDC *Morbidity and Mortality Weekly Report* (*MMWR*) 67, no. 45 (November 16, 2018): 1276–77. https://www.cdc.gov/mmwr/volumes/67/wr/mm6745a5.htm?s_cid=mm6745a5_w.

Cultural Survival Inc. "Huichol." *Cultural Survival Quarterly Magazine*. June 1992. https://www.culturalsurvival.org/publications/cultural-survival-quarterly/huichol.

Cyma Technologies (website). "Research Update on the Sound Techniques of Cymatechnologies: The Cyma 1000 Cymatechnologies Device Successfully Trialed on Thoroughbred Racehorses." https://cymatechnologies.com/sound-from-ancient-roots/sound-therapy-articles/research-update-on-the-sound-techniques-of-cymatechnologies.

Dance for PD (website). "About Us." https://danceforparkinsons.org/about-the-program.

"Dancing Can Reverse the Signs of Aging in the Brain." *ScienceDaily* 25 (August 2017). www.sciencedaily.com/releases/2017/08/170825124902.htm.

"Decline of the Colosseum." http://www.tribunesandtriumphs.org/colosseum/decline-of-the-colosseum.htm.

Delzo, Janissa. "Improve Brain Function by Playing Super Mario and Other Video Games, Science Says." *Newsweek* online. December 7, 2017, 4:23 p.m. http://www.newsweek.com/improve-brain-function-playing-super-mario-and-other-video-games-science-says-741592.

Denchak, Melissa. "Paris Climate Agreement: Everything You Need to Know." December 18, 2018. https://www.nrdc.org/stories/paris-climate-agreement-everything-you-need-know.

Deschamp, Justin. "HeartMath Institute: The Schumann Resonances Are Not Rising." May 13, 2017. http://www.stillnessinthestorm.com/2017/05/heartmath-institute-the-schumann-resonances-are-not-increasing.html.

Devinsky, Orrin, J. Helen Cross, Linda Laux, J. Helen Cross, and Eric Marsh. "Trial of Cannabidiol for Drug-Resistant Seizures in the Dravet Syndrome." *New England Journal of Medicine* 376 (May 25, 2017): 2011–2020. Accessed online at http://www.nejm.org/doi/10.1056/NEJMoa1611618.

Deyhle, Annette, "Earth's Atmosphere, Schumann Resonance, and the Ionosphere." https://www.heartmath.org/gci-commentaries/earths-atmosphere-schumann-resonance-and-the-ionosphere/.

Dispenza, Joe. *Becoming Supernatural: How Common People Are Doing the Uncommon.* Carlsbad, CA: Hay House, 2017.

Dodds, Lance, and Zachary Dodds. "The Sober Truth: Debunking the Bad Science behind the 12-Step Program and the Rehab Industry." http://sobertruthbook.com/.

Dong, Paul, and Aristide H. Esser. *Chi Gong: The Ancient Chinese Way to Health.* St. Paul, MN: Paragon House, 1990.

Duffy, Thomas P. "The Flexner Report—100 Years Later." *Yale Journal of Biology and Medicine* 84, no. 3 (September 2011): 269–76. Published online September 2011. https://www.ncbi.nlm.nih.gov/pmc/articles/PMC3178858/.

Eagle, Joshua. "3 Powerful Tools for Pineal Gland Activation." https://wakeup-world.com/2015/04/04/the-3-most-powerful-tools-for-pineal-gland-activation/.

Edelstein, Emma J., and Ludwig Edelstein. *Asclepius: Interpretation of the Testimonies.* Reprint. Baltimore: Johns Hopkins University Press, 1998. https://jhupbooks.press.jhu.edu/content/asclepius.

Editors at Chopra.com. "Shakti: A Universal Force." https://chopra.com/article/shakti-universal-force.

El-Seedi, H. R., P. A. De Smet, O. Beck, G. Possnert, and J. G. Bruhn. "Prehistoric Peyote Use: Alkaloid Analysis and Radiocarbon Dating of Archaeological Specimens of *Lophophroa* from Texas." *Journal of Ethnopharmacology* 101, no. 1–3 (October 3, 2005): 238–242. Sourced at https://www.sciencedirect.com/science/article/pii/S0378874105002990.

Emoto, Masaru. *The Secret Life of Water.* Atria paperback/Simon & Schuster, 2005.

English Heritage website. "History of Stonehenge." https://www.english-heritage.org.uk/visit/places/stonehenge/history-and-stories/history/.

____. "Research on Stonehenge." http://www.english-heritage.org.uk/visit/places/stonehenge/history/research/.

Environmental News Network Staff. "Dolphins Studied for Pollution's Impact." February 4. 1999. http://www.cnn.com/TECH/science/9902/04/dolphins.enn/.

Epel, E. S., E. H. Blackburn, J. Lin, F. S. Dhabhar N. E. Adler, J. D. Morrow, and R. M. Cawthon. "Accelerated Telomere Shortening in Response to Life Stress." *Proceedings of the National Academy of Sciences of the United States of America* 101, no. 49 (2004): 17312–17315. https://www.ncbi.nlm.nih.gov/pmc/articles/PMC534658/.

Epel, E., J. Daubenmier, J. T. Moskowitz, S. Folkman, and E. Blackburn. "Can Meditation Slow Rate of Cellular Aging? Cognitive Stress, Mindfulness, and Telomeres." *Annals of the New York Academy of Sciences* 1172 (August 2009): 34–53. doi: 10.1111/j.1749-6632.2009.04414.x.

Espuig, Maria Dasi. "Stonehenge Secrets Revealed by Underground Map." BBC News (September 10, 2014). https://www.bbc.com/news/science-environment-29126854.

Euclid. "Euclid's *Elements*." Book VI. Definition 3. https://mathcs.clarku.edu/~djoyce/elements/bookVI/defVI3.html.

Facts and Details (website). "Rumi and the Whirling Dervishes." http://factsanddetails.com/world/cat55/sub394/item1436.html.

Ferguson, J. M. "SSRI Antidepressant Medications: Adverse Effects and Tolerability." *Primary Care Companion to The Journal of Clinical Psychiatry* 3, no. 1 (2001): 22–27.

Finley, Bruce. "It's Not Your Imagination: More Trees Than Ever Are Standing Dead in Colorado Forests." February 15, 2017. https://www.denverpost.com/2017/02/15/dead-trees-colorado-forests/.

Fournier, Jay C., Robert J. DeRubeis, Steven D. Hollon, S. Dimidjian, J. D. Amsterdam, R. C. Shelton, and J. Fawcett. "Antidepressant Drug Effects and Depression Severity: A Patient-Level Meta-analysis." *Journal of the American Medical Association* 303, no. 1 (2010): 47–53. https://doi.org/10.1001/jama.2009.1943.

Garilli, Bianca. "MTHFR Mutation: A Missing Piece in the Chronic Disease Puzzle." June 2012. https://holisticprimarycare.net/topics/topics-a-g/functional-medicine/1353-mthfr-mutation-a-missing-piece-in-the-chronic-disease-puzzle.html.

Gefter, Amanda. "Is the Universe a Fractal?" *New Scientist* online. March 7, 2007. https://www.newscientist.com/article/mg19325941-600-is-the-universe-a-fractal/.

Gillam, Carey. "Roundup Herbicide Research Shows Plant, Soil Problems." https://www.reuters.com/article/us-glyphosate/roundup-herbicide-research-shows-plant-soil-problems-idUSTRE77B58A20110812.

Gilmor, T. M. "The Tomatis Method and the Genesis of Listening." *Journal of Prenatal & Perinatal Psychology & Health* 4, no. 1 (1989): 9–26.

Global Consciousness Project. "Introduction to GCP." http://noosphere.princeton.edu/gcpintro.html.

Goldman, Jonathan. "The Humming Effect: The Simplest Sound Is the Most Profound." August 17, 2017. https://www.soundhealersassociation.org/blog/139-the-humming-effect-the-simplest-sound-is-the-most-profound-2017-by-jonathan-goldman.html.

____. *The 7 Secrets of Sound Healing.* rev. ed. Carlsbad, CA: Hay House, 2008.

Goldman, Jonathan, and Andi Goldman. *The Humming Effect: Sound Healing for Health and Happiness.* Rochester VT: Healing Arts Press, 2017.

Greek Islands Post Cards (website). "The Kos Castle of the Knights." http://www.greekisland.co.uk/kos/sights/knights-castle.html.

Grey, Alex. "Alex Grey Quotations." https://www.quotetab.com/quotes/by-alex-grey#gLOGDqbMByMbx0WS.97.

Griffiths, Roland R., W. Richards, M. Johnson, U. McCann, and R. Jesse. "Mystical-Type Experiences Occasioned by Psilocybin Mediate the Attribution of Personal Meaning and Spiritual Significance 14 Months Later." *Journal of Psychopharmacology* 22, no. 6 (August 2008): 621–63, https://doi.org/10.1177/0269881108094300. Sourced at http://journals.sagepub.com/doi/abs/10.1177/0269881108094300?url_ver=Z39.88-2003&rfr_id=ori:rid:crossref.org&rfr_dat=cr_pub%3dpubmed.

Griffiths, Roland R., W. A. Richards, Una D. McCann, and R. Jesse, "Psilocybin Can Occasion Mystical Type Experiences Having Substantial and Sustained Personal Meaning and Spiritual Significance." *Psychopharmacology* 187, no. 3 (August 2006): 268–83, https://doi.org/ doi: 10.1007/s00213-006-0457-5.

Griffiths, Roland R., M. W. Johnson, M. A. Carducci, A. Umbricht, W. A. Richards, B. D. Richards, M. P. Cosimano, M. A. Klinedinst. "Psilocybin Produces Substantial and Sustained Decreases in Depression and Anxiety in Patients with Life-threatening Cancer: A Randomized Double-blind Trial." *Journal of Psychopharmacology* 30, no. 12 (2016): 1181–97, http://journals.sagepub.com/doi/pdf/10.1177/0269881116675513.

Grof, Stanislav and Christina. *Holotropic Breathwork: A New Approach to Self-Exploration and Therapy.* Albany: State University of New York Press, 2010.

Grof Transpersonal Training (website). "About Holotropic Breathwork." http://www.holotropic.com/holotropic-breathwork/about-holotropic-breathwork/.

Gun Violence Archive. "Gun Violence Archives: Past Summary Ledgers— Archives 2014–2018." http://www.gunviolencearchive.org/past-tolls.

Gupta, Sanjay. "Weed 4: Pot vs. Pills: Dr. Sanjay Gupta Reports." CNN Special Report. CNN transcript of April 29, 2018. http://transcripts. cnn.com/TRANSCRIPTS/1804/29/se.01.html.

Gupta, Subash C., Sridevi Patchva, and Bharat B. Aggarwal. "Therapeutic Roles of Curcumin: Lessons Learned from Clinical Trials." *Journal of the American Association of Pharmaceutical Scientists* 15, no. 1 (January 2013): 195–218. Published online November 10, 2012. Sourced at https://www.ncbi.nlm.nih.gov/pmc/articles/PMC3535097/.

Hall, Stephen S. "Hidden Treasures in Junk DNA." October 1, 2012. Originally published with the title "Journey to the Genetics Interior." Sourced at *Scientific American* online. https://www.scientificamerican. com/article/hidden-treasures-in-junk-dna.

Hammond, Holly. "The Timeline and History of Yoga in America." *Yoga Journal* online. (August 29, 2007). http://yogajournal.com/yoga-101/ yogas-trip-america.

Hancock, Graham. *Heaven's Mirror: Quest for the Lost Civilization.* Manhattan: Three Rivers Press, 1998.

Haramein, Nassim. Facebook page. https://www.facebook.com/Nassim. Haramein.official/. February 12, 2018, at 3:22 p.m.

___. "The I-Ching Encodes the Geometry of the Fabric of Space-Time." https://www.facebook.com/Nassim.Haramein.official/videos/286050751586190/.

Hart, Francene. *Sacred Geometry of Nature: Journey on the Path of the Divine.* Rochester, VT: Bear & Co., 2017.

HeartMath Institute website. "Researching the Human Heart and Brain." https://www.heartmath.org/research/.

Herper, Matthew (Forbes staff). "David Graham on the Vioxx Verdict." August 19, 2005. https://www.forbes.com/2005/08/19/merck-vioxx-graham_cx_mh_0819graham.html#7251a0835698.

Hill, David. "Peru's Ayahuasca Industry Booms as Westerners Search for Alternative Healing." January 7, 2016. https://www.theguardian.com/travel/2016/jun/07/peru-ayahuasca-drink-boom-amazon-spirituality-healing.

Hipskind, S. G., F. L Grover Jr., T. R. Fort, D. Helffenstein, T. J. Burke, S. A. Quint, G. Bussiere G, M. Stone, T. Hurtado. "Pulsed Transcranial Red/Near-Infrared Light Therapy Using Light-Emitting Diodes Improves Cerebral Blood Flow and Cognitive Function in Veterans with Chronic Traumatic Brain Injury: A Case Series." *Journal of Photomedicine and Laser Surgery.* November 28, 2018. http://doi.org/10.1089/pho.2018.4489.

"History of Kos." After S. Rossiter, *Blue Guide Greece*, London, 1977. Sourced at https://www.ostia-antica.org/kos/history/history.htm.

History Wiz. "Asclepius and the Temples of Healing." http://www.historywiz.com/didyouknow/asclepius.html.

Hoffmann, Albert. *LSD: My Problem Child—Reflections on Sacred Drugs, Mysticism and Science.* New York: McGraw-Hill, 1980.

——. *Rational Mysticism.* Boston: Mariner Books, 2004.

Hunter, Richard G. "Epigenetic Effects of Stress and Corticosteroids in the Brain." *Frontiers in Cellular Neuroscience* 6 (2012):18.

Innovative Biophysical Technologies. "Original Research Discoveries" (of Glen Rhine). http://www.innobioteck.com/discoveries.html.

International Hippocratic Foundation of Kos. "History." http://hippocratic-foundation.org/the-institution/history.

Jacobs, Andrew. "Opposition to Breast-Feeding Resolution by U.S. Stuns World Health Officials." July 8, 2018. https://www.nytimes.com/2018/07/08/health/world-health-breastfeeding-ecuador-trump.html.

Jacobs, T. L., E. S. Epel, J. Lin, E. H. Blackburn, O. M. Wolkowitz, D. A. Bridwell, A. P. Zanesco, S. R. Aichele, B. K. Sahdra, K. A. MacLean, B. G. King, P. R. Shaver, E. L. Roenberg, E. Ferrer, B. A. Wallace, C. D. Saron. "Intensive Meditation Training, Immune Cell Telomerase Activity, and Psychological Mediators." *Psychoneuroendocrinology* 36, no. 5 (June 2011): 664–81.

Jenkins, J. S., "The Mozart Effect." *Journal of the Royal Society of Music* 94, no. 4 (April 2001): 170–72). Sourced at https://www.ncbi.nlm.nih.gov/pmc/articles/PMC1281386/.

Jeschke, Mark. "Weed Management in the Era of Glyphosate Resistance." https://www.pioneer.com/home/site/us/agronomy/weed-mgmt-and-glyphosate-resis/.

Jiao, S. S., L. L. Shen, C. Zhu, X. L. Bu, Y. H. Liu, C. H. Liu, X. Q. Yao, L. L. Zhang, H. D. Zhou, D. G. Walker, J. Tan, J. Gotz, X. F. Zhou, and Y. J. Wang. "Brain-derived Neurotrophic Factor Protects against Tau-related Neurodegeneration of Alzheimer's Disease." *Translational Psychiatry* 6, no. 10 (October 4, 2016): e907. https://doi.org/10.1038/tp.2016.186.

Jouanna, Jacques. *Hippocrates.* Translated by Malcolm B. De Bevoise. Baltimore and London: Johns Hopkins University Press, 1999.

Jung, Carl. *Symbols and the Interpretation of Dreams.* Collected Works 18. Princeton: University Press, 1976.

Kalyani, Bangalore G., G. Venkatasubramanian, R. Arasappa, N. P. Rao, S. V. Kalmady, R. V. Behere, H. Rao M. K. Vasudev, B. N. Gangadhar. "Neurohemodynamic Correlates of 'Om' Chanting." *International Journal of Yoga* 4, no. 1 (2011): 3–6. dfhttp://yogafordepression.com/wp-content/uploads/Neurohemodynamic-correlates-of-'OM'-chanting.pdf.

Karp, Aaron. "Estimating Global Civilian-Held Firearms Numbers." Briefing Paper 2018. http://www.smallarmssurvey.org/fileadmin/docs/T-Briefing-Papers/SAS-BP-Civilian-Firearms-Numbers.pdf.

Kassewitz, Jack, Michael T. Hyson, John S. Reid, and Regina L. Barrera. "A Phenomenon Discovered While Imaging Dolphin Echolocation Sounds." *Journal of Marine Science: Research & Development.* July 15, 2016. https://www.omicsonline.org/open-access/a-phenomenon-discovered-while-imaging-dolphin-echolocation-sounds-2155-9910-1000202.php?aid=76570.

Kinsley, Austin. "Restorations at Stonehenge." Oct. 1, 2017. https://www.silentearth.org/restorations-at-stonehenge-2/.

Khaliya. "The Promise of Ecstasy for PTSD." *New York Times* op-ed. November 3, 2017. https://www.nytimes.com/2017/11/03/opinion/ecstasy-ptsd.html.

Khesbak, Hassan, Olesya Savchuk, Satoru Tsushima, and Karim Fahmy. "The Role of Water H-Bond Imbalances in B-DNA Substrate Transitions and Peptide Recognition Revealed by Time-Resolved FTIR Spectroscopy." *Journal of the American Chemical Society* 133, no. 15 (2011): 5834–42. https://doi.org/10.1021/ja108863v.

Klosin, Adam, Eduard Casas, Christina Hidalgo-Carcedo, Tanya Vavouri, and Ben Lehner. "Transgenerational Transmission of Environmental Information in C. Elegans." *Science* 356, no. 6335 (April 2017), 320–23. http://science.sciencemag.org/content/356/6335/320.full.

Kos Island, Greece (website). "Asclepeion of Kos." https://www.kos4all.com/4899/asclepeion-of-kos/.

Kotler, Stephen. "Exploring the Intersection between Radical Innovation, Peak Performance, & Disruptive Technology." http://www.stevenkotler.com/.

Kotler, Stephen, and Jamie Wheal. *Stealing Fire: How Silicon Valley, the Navy Seals, and Maverick Scientists Are Revolutionizing the Way We Live and Work.* New York: Dey Street Books, 2017.

Kumar, Shiv Basant, R. Yadav, R. K. Yadav, M Tolahumase, and R. Dada. "Telomerase Activity and Cellular Aging Might Be Positively Modified by a Yoga-Based Lifestyle Intervention." *The Journal of Alternative and Complementary Medicine* 21, no. 6 (June 2015): 370–72.

Kunz, Dieter, S. Schmitz, R. Mahlberg, A. Mohr, C. Stöter, K. J. Wolf, and W. M. Hermann. "A New Concept for Melatonin Deficit: on Pineal Calcification and Melatonin Excretion." *Neuropsychopharmacology* 21, no. 6 (January 2000): 765–72.

Lawlor, Robert. *Sacred Geometry: Philosophy & Practice.* London, UK/New York: Thames & Hudson, 1982.

Lee, Michelle Ye Hee. "The Missing Context behind the Widely Cited Statistic That There Are 22 Veteran Suicides a Day." https://www.washingtonpost.com/news/fact-checker/wp/2015/02/04/the-missing-context-behind-a-widely-cited-statistic-that-there-are-22-veteran-suicides-a-day/?noredirect=on&utm_term=.9ba6e5209fc2.

Lees-Milne, James. *Saint Peter's—The Story of Saint Peter's Basilica in Rome.* London: Hamish Hamilton, 1967.

Leung, Hillary. "Stonehenge's Rocks Have Been Traced to Two Quarries 180 Miles Away." Updated Feb. 21, 2019. http://time.com/5534188/stonehenge-bluestone-quarries-180-miles-away/.

Lipton, Bruce. *The Biology of Belief: Unleashing the Power of Consciousness, Matter and Miracles.* 10th anniversary edition. Carlsbad, CA, 2016.

Loria, Kevin. "How Psychedelics like Psilocybin and LSD Actually Change the Way People See the World." *Business Insider.* February 26, 2017. https://www.businessinsider.com/a-new-understanding-film-shows-how-psilocybin-changes-perception-2017-2.

Luckman, Sol. "All Healing Is Really Self-Healing." https://www.tokenrock.com/articles/all-healing-is-really-self-healing/. Article adapted from the author's *Potentiate Your DNA: A Practical Guide to Healing & Transformation with the Regenetics Method.*

Luke, Jennifer. "Fluoride Deposition in the Aged Human Pineal Gland." *Caries Research* 35, no. 2 (2001): 125–28. (Official Journal of the European Organization for Caries Research.) Research has also shown a link between pineal gland calcification and Alzheimer's.

Luminet, Jean-Pierre, Jeffrey R. Weeks, Alain Riazuelo, Roland Lehoucq, and Jean-Philippe Uzan. "Dodecahedral Space Topology as an Explanation for Weak Wide-Angle Temperature Correlations in the Cosmic Microwave Background." *Nature* 425 (October 9, 2003): 593–95.

Lund University. "Dolphins Use Double Sonar: Researchers Discover That Dolphins Can Generate Two Sound Beam Projections Simultaneously." *ScienceDaily* June 8, 2011. www.sciencedaily.com/releases/2011/06/110607112338.htm. Journal reference. https://doi.org/10.1098/rsbl.2011.0396.

Mandrake, K. *The Psilocybin Mushroom Bible: The Definitive Guide to Growing and Using Magic Mushrooms.* San Francisco: Green Candy Press, 2016.

MAPS. "A Phase 3 Program of MDMA-Assisted Psychotherapy for the Treatment of Severe Posttraumatic Stress Disorder (PTSD)." https://maps.org/research/mdma/ptsd/phase3.

Marketos, Spyros G. "History of Medicine." http://asclepieion.mpl.uoa.gr/Parko/marketos2.htm.

Markey, Sean. "CBD Bioavailability: What's the Best Way to Absorb CBD?" July 31, 2018, updated October 19. https://www.cannahealth.org/cbd-bioavailability-whats-the-best-way-to-absorb-cbd/.

Marsh, Adam G., Matthew T. Cottrell, and Morton F. Goldman. "Epigenetic DNA Methylation Profiling with MSRE: A Quantitative NGS Approach Using a Parkinson's Disease Test Case." *Frontiers in Genetics* (November 2, 2016). https://doi.org/10.3389/fgene.2016.00191.

Martin-Ruiz, Carmen, Heather O. Dickinson, Barbara Keys, Elise Rowan, Rose Anne Kenney, Thomas Von Zglinicki. "Telomere Length Predicts Poststroke Mortality, Dementia, and Cognitive Decline." *Annals of Neurology* (May 9, 2006). https://doi.org/10.1002/ana.20869. Abstract: http://onlinelibrary.wiley.com/doi/10.1002/ana.20869/abstract.

Master Teacher. "Drug Harm Charts and Psychedelics." Cognitive Liberty—UK. August 9, 2011. https://cognitivelibertyuk.wordpress. com/2011/08/09/drug-harm-charts-psychedelics.

Mayo Clinic Staff. "Selective Serotonin Reuptake Inhibitors (SSRIs)." May 17, 2018. https://www.mayoclinic.org/diseases-conditions/depression/ in-depth/ssris/art-20044825.

McCraty, Rollin, Mike Atkinson, and Dana Tomasino. "Modulation of DNA Conformation by Heart-Focused Intention." http://www.aipro.info/ drive/File/224.pdf.

McFarlane, Thomas J. "Quantum Physics, Depth Psychology, and Beyond" (February 26, 2000, rev. June 21, 2000). http://www.integralscience. org/psyche-physis.html.

McKenna, Terence. *The Stoned Ape Theory.* https://www.youtube.com/ watch?v=ZnEKoFrx1rI.

McKie, Robin. "Interview—Colin Blakemore: How the Human Brain Got Bigger by Accident and Not Through Evolution." https://www.the-guardian.com/technology/2010/mar/28/colin-blakemore-how-human-brains-got-bigger.

Meisner, Gary B. "Life/DNA Spiral as a Golden Section." http://www.golden-number.net/dna/.

___. " Life/Human Hand and Foot." http://www.goldennumber.net/human-hand-foot/.

___. "Phi/What is the Fibonacci Sequence (aka Fibonacci Series)?" https:// www.goldennumber.net/fibonacci-series/.

Meyer, J. S. "3,4—Methylenedioxymethamphetamine (MDMA): Current Perspectives." *Substance Abuse and Rehabilitation* 4 (November 21, 2013): 83–99.

Mohata, Vandana. "Mantras: An Interview with Jonathan Goldman." https:// www.healingsounds.com/mantras-an-interview-with-jonathan-goldman/.

Monroe Institute. https://www.monroeinstitute.org/.

Monteverde Travel Guide (website). "Monteverde, Costa Rica." http://www.monteverdeinfo.com/.

Morales, Klaus, and Tulio Vinicius. "Amazon Rainforest: Biodiversity and Biopiracy." *STUDENT BMJ* (*British Medical Journal*) 13 (2003): 386–87. Source for number of Amazon plant species. http://student.bmj.com/student/view-article.html?id=sbmj0510386.

Myss, Caroline. "The Seven Chakras." https://www.myss.com/free-resources/world-religions/hinduism/the-seven-chakras/.

Narby, Jeremy. *The Cosmic Serpent: DNA and the Origins of Knowledge.* Los Angeles: Jeremy P. Tarcher/Putman, now the Tarcher Perigee imprint of New York: Penguin Random House, 1998.

National Aeronautics and Space Administration (NASA) online. "Imagine the Universe: Objects of Interest: The Milky Way Galaxy." Updated December 2015. https://imagine.gsfc.nasa.gov/science/objects/milkyway1.html.

National Institute of Health (NIH). "Alcohol Facts and Statistics." https://www.niaaa.nih.gov/alcohol-health/overview-alcohol-consumption/alcohol-facts-and-statistics.

____. "Prescription Opioid Use Is a Risk Factor for Heroin Use." https://www.drugabuse.gov/publications/research-reports/relationship-between-prescription-drug-heroin-abuse/prescription-opioid-use-risk-factor-heroin-use.

National Institute on Drug Abuse (NIDA). "Overdose Death Rates." Rev. January 2019. https://www.drugabuse.gov/related-topics/trends-statistics/overdose-death-rates._

New World Encyclopedia contributors. "Luca Pacioli." *New World Encyclopedia.* http://www.newworldencyclopedia.org/p/index.php?title=Luca_Pacioli&oldid=1013453. Revision as of 15:37, August 2, 2018, by Rosie Tanabe; they drew as well from "Luca Pacioli," Wikipedia.

New York Times obituary. "Dr. Albert Einstein Dies in Sleep at 76: World Mourns Loss of Great Scientist." April 19, 1955. https://archive.nytimes.com/www.nytimes.com/learning/general/onthisday/bday/0314.html.

Nichols, Wallace J., *Blue Mind: The Surprising Science That Shows How Being Near, In, On, or Underwater Can Make You Happier, Healthier, More Connected, and Better at What You Do.* New York City: Little Brown and Co., 2014.

Nicolae, Chiriac C., and Alina Dragomir. "Dacians and the Great Sanctuary at Sarmizegetusa/the Dacian Calendar." March 5, 2018. https://www.matrixdisclosure.com/dacians-sanctuary-sarmizegetusa-calendar/.

Novotney, Amy. "Music as Medicine." *American Psychologist* 44, no. 10 (November 2013), 46. Sourced at American Psychological Association website. http://www.apa.org/monitor/2013/11/music.aspx.

Nutton, Vivian. *Ancient Medicine.* 2nd ed. New York: Routledge, 2013.

O'Brien, Barbara. "Mount Meru in Buddhist Mythology." Updated July 24, 2017. https://www.thoughtco.com/mount-meru-449900.

Organic Consumers Association. "Monsanto Is Putting Normal Seeds Out of Reach." https://www.organicconsumers.org/news/monsanto-putting-normal-seeds-out-reach.

Orlic, Christian. "The Origins of Directed Panspermia." January 9, 2013. https://blogs.scientificamerican.com/guest-blog/the-origins-of-directed-panspermia/.

Osborn, David K. "Greek Medicine." https://www.organicconsumers.org/news/monsanto-putting-normal-seeds-out-reach.

PandoraStar. "The Experience." https://pandorastar.co.uk/introduction/.

Pappas, Stephanie. "Human Body Part That Stumped Leonardo da Vinci Revealed." https://www.livescience.com/20157-anatomy-drawings-leonardo-da-vinci.html.

Pearson, Mike Parker, Josh Pollard, Colin Richards, Kate Welham. "Megalith Quarries for Stonehenge's Bluestones." *Antiquity* 93, nr. 367 (February 2019): 45–62. https://doi.org/10.15184/aqy.2018.111.

Pesticide Action Network North America (website). "Monsanto Merger . . . or Bust?" http://www.panna.org/blog/monsanto-merger-or-bust.

Petri, G., P. Expert, F. Turkheimer, R. Carhart-Harris, D. Nutt, P. J. Hellyer, and F. Vaccarino. "Homological Scaffolds of Brain Functional Networks." December 6, 2014. https://doi.org/10.1098/rsif.2014.0873.

Plans, David. "We've lost Touch with Our Bodies." February 5, 2019. https://blogs.scientificamerican.com/observations/weve-lost-touch-with-our-bodies.

Plummer, Gordon. *The Mathematics of the Cosmic Mind.* Quoted by Robert Lawlor. *Sacred Geometry.* 1982. Sourced in the article "309ct 3-D20-Icosahedron-Real Amethyst Quartz Gemstone #213." https://rjrockshop.com/products/309ct-3-d20-icosahedron-real-amethyst-quartz-gemstone-hand-carved-213?variant=581238685709.

Pollan, Michael. *How to Change Your Mind: What the New Science of Psychedelics Teaches Us about Consciousness, Dying, Addiction, Depression, and Transcendence.* New York: Penguin Press, 2018.

Powers, Richard. "Dancing Makes You Smarter." https://socialdance.stanford. edu/syllabi/smarter.htm.

Princeton University. "Imaging in Living Cells Reveals How 'Junk DNA' Switches On a Gene: Video shows DNA enhancers finding and activating a target gene in a living cell." *ScienceDaily* July 23, 2018. http:// www.sciencedaily.com/releases/2018/07/180723142817.htm. Original article. https://doi.org/10.1038/s41588-018-0175-z.

"Puakai: Healing through the Energy of Mother Nature (website). https:// puakaihealing.com/model/.

"Rainforest Facts: The Disappearing Rainforests." http://www.rain-tree. com/facts.htm#.WmONzWcY7BU. Some material on this webpage is excerpted from Leslie Taylor. *The Healing Power of Rainforest Herbs.* Garden City, NY: SquareOne Publishers, 2004.

Rauscher, F. H., and G. L. Shaw. "Key Components of the Mozart Effect." *Perceptual and Motor Skills.* June 1, 1998. Sourced at http://journals. sagepub.com/doi/abs/10.2466/pms.1998.86.3.835.

Rauscher, F. H., G. L. Shaw, and Katherine N. Ky. "Music and Spatial Task Performance." *Nature* 365 (October 14, 1993): 611 (research article that spawned the Mozart-effect book). Available online at https://www.nature.com/articles/365611a0.

Rauscher, Frances H., Gordan L. Shaw, Linda J. Levine, Katherine N. Ky. "Music and Spatial Task Performance: A Causal Relationship." Presented at the American Psychological Association 102nd Annual Convention. Los Angeles, CA. August 12–16, 1994. Sourced at http://www.burch-school.com/music-and-spatial-task-performance-a-causal-relationship/.

Regueiro, Javier. *San Pedro Huachuma: Opening the Pathways of the Heart.* 2nd ed. Las Vegas: Lifestyle Entrepreneurs Press, 2017.

Rehfeld, Kathrin, Patrick Müller, Norman Aye, Marlen Schmicker, Milos Dordevic, Jörn Kufmann, Anita Hökelmann, and Notger G. Möller. "Dancing or Fitness Sport? The Effects of Two Training Programs on Hippocampal Plasticity and Balance Abilities in Healthy Seniors." *Frontiers in Human Neuroscience* 11 (June 15, 2017): 305. Accessed online at "Dancing Can Reverse the Signs of Aging in the Brain," *ScienceDaily* 25 (August 2017). www.sciencedaily.com/re-leases/2017/08/170825124902.htm.

Reid, Annaliese, and John Stuart. "Sound Healing—Ancient Sounds." https:// www.tokenrock.com/sound_healing/sounds_of_the_ancients/. Content courtesy of the Reids, © 2011. http://www.cymascope.com.

Reid, John Stuart. Email to the author March 14, 2019.

Reid, John Stuart, Annaliese Reid, Vera Gadman, and James Stuart Reid. "Cymatics Research—Biology." https://www.cymascope.com/cyma_research/biology.html.

——. "First 'What-the-dolphin-saw' Image of a Submerged Man: Cymatic-Holographic Imaging Technique." http://www.cymascope.com/cyma_research/oceanography.html.

——. "Welcome to Our Cymatics Research." https://www.cymascope.com/cyma_research/index.html.

Rein, Glen. "Effect of Conscious Intention on Human DNA." *Proceedings of the International Forum on New Science.* Denver, CO. October 1996. https://www.item-bioenergy.com/infocenter/ConsciousIntentiononDNA.pdf.

Reuters (NBC News). "Bernie Sanders Asks Why Drug, Once Free, Now Costs $375,000." February 4, 2019. https://www.nbcnews.com/politics/2020-election/bernie-sanders-asks-why-drug-once-free-now-costs-375-n966746.

Rossi, Andrea, A. Molinaro, E. Savi, S. Micheletti, J. Galli, G. Chirico, and E. Fazzi. "Music Reduces Pain Perception in Healthy Newborns: A Comparison between Different Music Tracks and Recorded Heartbeat." *Early Human Development* 124 (2018): 7–10.

"Secret of Water—The Movie." www.secretofwaterthemovie.com.

"So Sound Solutions." http://www.sosoundsolutions.com/products/so-sound-treatment-tables.

Rodriguez, Tori. "Descendants of Holocaust Survivors Have Altered Stress Hormones." March 1, 2015. https://www.scientificamerican.com/article/descendants-of-holocaust-survivors-have-altered-stress-hormones/.

Roman Empire & Colosseum (website). "Decline of the Colosseum." http://www.tribunesandtriumphs.org/colosseum/decline-of-the-colosseum.htm.

Rowe, Aaron. "Diamonds 'Entangled' in Physics Feat." CNN online. December 7, 2011. http://lightyears.blogs.cnn.com/2011/12/07/diamonds-entangled-in-physics-feat/.

"Rumi and the Whirling Dervishes." Facts and Details. http://factsanddetails.com/world/cat55/sub394/item1436.html.

Salk Institute website. "Cannabinoids Remove Plaque-forming Alzheimer's Proteins from Brain Cells: Preliminary Lab Studies at the Salk Institute Find THC Reduces Beta Amyloid Proteins in Human Neurons." June

27, 2016. https://www.salk.edu/news-release/cannabinoids-remove-plaque-forming-alzheimers-proteins-from-brain-cells/.

Saunders, N. J. *Animal Spirits*. London: Duncan Baird Publishers, 1995.

Schultes, Richard Evans (1938). "The Appeal of Peyote (*Lophophora Williamsii*) as a Medicine." *American Anthropologist* 40, no. 4, Part 1 (1938): 698–715. Online: http://www.samorini.it/doc1/alt_aut/sz/schultes_pey.htm.

Schultes, Richard Evans, and Albert Hofmann. "The Tracks of the Little Deer." From Plants of the Gods: *Their Sacred, Healing and Hallucinogenic Powers*. Vermont: Healing Arts Press, 1992. https://www.peyote.org/.

Seaburn, Paul. "The Return of the Stone Ape Theory of Evolution." July 27, 2017. http://mysteriousuniverse.org/2017/07/the-return-of-the-stoned-ape-theory-of-evolution/.

Shammas, Masood A. "Telomeres, Lifestyle, Cancer, and Aging." https://www.ncbi.nlm.nih.gov/pmc/articles/PMC3370421/.

Shane, Leo III, and Patricia Kime. "New VA Study Finds 20 Veterans Commit Suicide Each Day." *Military Times*. https://www.militarytimes.com/veterans/2016/07/07/new-va-study-finds-20-veterans-commit-suicide-each-day/.

Shaw, Edwina. "Science Shows Dolphins Communicate Holographically." December 1, 2016. https://upliftconnect.com/dolphins-communicate-holographically/.

Shulgin, Alexander, and Ann Shulgin. *Tihkal*, Berkeley: Transform Press, 1997.

Silva, Freddy. The Prophets Conference. http://www.greatmystery.org/nl/salisbury09geometry.html.

Sircus, Mark. "Carpet Bombing Cancer with Invincible Oxygen." February 11, 2014. http://drsircus.com/general/carpet-bombing-cancer-with-invincible-oxygen.

Smith, B. Sidney. "Fibonacci Sequence." *Platonic Realms Interactive Mathematics Encyclopedia*. March 1, 2013. Web: February 7, 2019. http://platonic-realms.com/encyclopedia/Fibonacci-sequence.

Smith, Patrick. "What Is the Legality of Ayahuasca in Your Home?" January 18, 2017. https://thethirdwave.co/legality-ayahuasca/.

Strassman, Rick J. *DMT: The Spirit Molecule. A Doctor's Revolutionary Research into the Biology of Near-Death and Mystical Experiences*. Rochester, VT: Park Street, 2001.

Subramanian, Sankara. "Adumu: The Traditional Maasai Dance." October 5,

2012. https://www.beontheroad.com/2012/10/adumu-traditional-maa-sai-dance.html#.

Swanson, Jerry W., MD. "Vitamin D and MS: Is There Any Connection?" http://www.mayoclinic.org/diseases-conditions/multiple-sclerosis/expert-answers/vitamin-d-and-ms/faq-20058258.

Tayag, Yasmin. "On 'Bicycle Day,' Albert Hofmann Took the First LSD Trip." April 19, 2017. https://www.inverse.com/article/14503-bicycle-day-albert-hofmann-lsd-acid-trip.

Taylor, John Maxwell. *Eros Ascending: The Life Transforming Power of Sacred Sexuality.* North Atlantic Books, 2009

Token Rock (website). "Flower of Life." http://www.tokenrock.com/explain-flower-of-life-46.html.

Tolle, Eckhart. *A New Earth: Awakening to Your Life's Purpose.* Reprint edition. New York: Penguin, 2008.

Tomatis (website). "Alfred Tomatis" under "Discover." https://www.tomatis.com/en.

Trafton, Anne. "Unique Visual Stimulation May Be New Treatment for Alzheimer's." http://news.mit.edu/2016/visual-stimulation-treatment-alzheimer-1207.

Ueshiba, Morihei. *The Art of Peace.* Translated and edited by John Stevens. Reprint. Boulder: Shambhala Pocket Library Series, 2018.

University of Idaho website. "The American Indian Religious Freedom Act 1978." http://www.webpages.uidaho.edu/~rfrey/329AIRFA.htm.

University of Leicester Press office. "Scientists Solve Riddle of Celestial Archaeology." March 27, 2014. http://www.astronomy.com/news/2014/03/scientists-solve-riddle-of-celestial-archaeology.

Unschuld, Paul U. *Medicine in China: A History of Ideas.* Berkeley: University of California Press, 1985.

Vaults of Erowid, The. "Walter Pahnke. January 18, 1931–July 10, 1971." https://erowid.org/culture/characters/pahnke_walter/pahnke_walter.shtml.

Verghese, Joe, Richard B. Lipton, Mindy J. Katz, Charles B. Hall, Carol A. Derby, Gail Kuslansky, Anne F. Ambrose, Martin Sliwinski, and Herman Buschke. "Leisure Activities and the Risk of Dementia in the Elderly." *New England Journal of Medicine* 348 (June 19, 2003): 2508–16. https://doi.org/10.1056/NEJMoa022252.

Vitruvius. *De Architectura.* Book V. Chapter 4.8. http://www.vitruvius.be/boek5h4.htm.

Wezit Research Group. "A Flickering Light." http://www.clinic.visnsoft.com/video1.htm.

Wheeling, Kate. "Bio Tech Company Marks Up Drug Cost by 5,000 Percent Because It Can." September 22, 2015. https://psmag.com/economics/biotech-company-marks-up-drug-cost-by-5000-percent-because-it-can.

Wikipedia. "Cyparissus."

Wikipedia. "Francisco Hernández de Toledo."

Wikipedia. *"Guns, Germs, and Steel."*

Wikipedia. "Luca Pacioli."

Wikipedia. "Sacred Geometry." "Plutarch attributed the belief to Plato, writing that Plato said god geometrizes continually." (*Convivialium disputationum,* liber 8,2).

Wikipedia. "World Population."

Wilton, Pete. "Vibration Rocks for Entangled Diamonds." December 16, 2011. https://phys.org/news/2011-12-vibration-entangled-diamonds.html#jC.p.

Winn, Michael. "Curing Cancer Naturally with Chi Kung [Qigong] Self-Healing Therapy." http://www.healingcancernaturally.com/medical-qigong-cancer-therapy.html.

Wolchover, Natalie. "A Jewel at the Heart of Quantum Physics." https://www.quantamagazine.org/20130917-a-jewel-at-the-heart-of-quantum-physics/.

Yogananda, Paramahansa (website). "Excerpts from *God Talks with Arjuna: The Bhagavad Gita* by Paramahansa Yogananda." http://yogananda.com.au/gita/gita0614om.html.

Young, Gloria A. "Sun Dance." Encyclopedia of Oklahoma History and Culture. The Oklahoma Historical Society. http://www.okhistory.org/publications/enc/entry.php?entry=SU008.

Illustrations

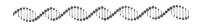

Illustrations

Illustrations

About the Author

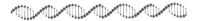

Fred Grover Jr., M.D., is a board-certified family physician, a Fellow of the American Academy of Family Physicians, whose practice focuses on preventative, functional, integrative, regenerative, and personalized medicine. He has additional board certifications in Integrative Medicine and Anti-Aging and Regenerative Medicine. Supporting healing in the deepest way, he emphasizes mindfulness-based practices in stress reduction, lifestyle, and nutrition to proactively promote wellness and reduce acute and chronic illness. He even has two rooms dedicated to meditation and sound healing in his medical office in Denver. He is also an Assistant Clinical Professor of Family Medicine at the University of Colorado and regularly teaches medical students and residents in the Integrative Medicine elective. His most recent research publication, in the November 2018 *Journal of Photomedicine and Laser Surgery*, demonstrated the benefits of transcranial near-infrared light therapy for the treatment of traumatic brain injury in veterans.

His adventurous world travels, coupled with passionate interest in spirituality, mindfulness, and health, have helped him discover healing beyond a prescription pad, leading him to understand unique ways of maintaining the expression of healthy DNA, while helping others do the same.